Endometriosis Relief Roadmap

Evidence-Based Practical Guide to
Diagnosis, Treatment, Surgery & Fertility

Joyce Eleanor Spears

ISBN: 978-1-7642608-7-9

Table of Contents

Chapter 1: What is Endometriosis

Sarah from Nairobi collapsed in her classroom at fifteen. The pain hit her like a lightning bolt straight through her abdomen, so severe that her teachers thought she was dying. "They were terrified," she recalls. "One teacher actually said she couldn't handle watching a student die in her hands." Seven and a half years later, after countless dismissive doctors and being told it was "just bad periods," Sarah finally got her answer: endometriosis.

Meanwhile, in Manchester, Emma spent her twenties being told she was "too sensitive" and needed to "toughen up." The UK's National Health Service sent her home with painkillers time after time. Twenty-seven years. That's how long it took for someone to take her pain seriously enough to investigate properly. By then, the endometriosis had spread so extensively that it had fused several of her organs together.

And in Houston, Texas, Maria's story echoes the same frustrating pattern. Despite having excellent private health insurance, she bounced between specialists for years. Gastroenterologists treated her for IBS. Psychiatrists prescribed antidepressants for her "stress-related" symptoms. Urologists ran test after test. Nobody connected the dots until a desperate emergency room visit at age thirty-two finally led to the right diagnosis.

These aren't unusual stories. They're heartbreakingly typical.

The staggering scope of this condition

One hundred ninety million women worldwide live with endometriosis right now. That's roughly one in ten women of reproductive age, though recent research suggests the number might be even higher. This condition doesn't care about your income, your education level, or what country you call home. From rural villages in Kenya to penthouses in New York City, endometriosis affects women across every culture and socioeconomic background.

Now, here's the thing that really gets me: despite affecting as many women as diabetes, endometriosis remains shockingly misunderstood, underdiagnosed, and poorly treated. The average diagnostic delay sits at 7.5 years globally, though some regions see delays stretching to nearly three decades.

You might be reading this because you're one of the millions still searching for answers. Or maybe you've just received your diagnosis and you're trying to make sense of what happens next. Perhaps you're supporting someone you love through this condition. Wherever you're coming from, you need real information, practical strategies, and most importantly, validation that what you're experiencing is real.

Because it is real. Every single bit of it.

What exactly is endometriosis anyway?

Let me paint you a picture that'll stick with you. Think of endometriosis like weeds in a garden. Normally, the uterine lining stays where it belongs, like flowers in designated beds. But in endometriosis, that tissue starts growing outside the uterus, like weeds spreading into areas they shouldn't be.

Here's where it gets complicated—and painful. This wayward tissue still acts like it's inside the uterus. Every month, it responds to your hormonal cycles, thickening and trying to shed. But unlike the tissue inside your uterus that can exit your body during menstruation, this trapped tissue has nowhere to go. It bleeds internally, causing inflammation, scarring, and the formation of adhesions that can literally glue your organs together.

Actually, wait. That sounds terrifying when I put it that way. Let me back up a bit.

The tissue itself isn't exactly the same as your uterine lining—it's similar but not identical. Scientists call it "endometrial-like tissue," and while that might seem like a small distinction, it matters for understanding how the disease works and why certain treatments help while others don't.

Understanding the stages (or why your pain doesn't match your diagnosis)

Doctors classify endometriosis into four stages, and this is where our garden analogy really helps:

Stage 1 (Minimal): Think of this as a few small weeds popping up here and there. You might have small lesions or spots of endometrial tissue, mostly on the surface of organs.

Stage 2 (Mild): Now those weeds are spreading a bit more. There are more implants, and they might be starting to go slightly deeper.

Stage 3 (Moderate): The weeds are taking over significant portions of the garden. You've got many implants, and they're going deep. Adhesions are starting to form—imagine the weeds' roots tangling things together.

Stage 4 (Severe): The garden is overrun. Large, deep implants are everywhere, and extensive adhesions might be distorting your anatomy, pulling organs out of their normal positions.

But here's what drives me absolutely crazy about this staging system: it doesn't correlate with pain levels. At all. You can have Stage 1 endometriosis and be in agony, or Stage 4 and have relatively mild symptoms. The location matters far more than the amount. A tiny spot of endometriosis on a nerve can cause excruciating pain, while larger lesions in less sensitive areas might cause no symptoms at all (Vercellini et al., 2023).

This disconnect between staging and symptoms leads to one of the most frustrating aspects of endometriosis: being told your pain "shouldn't be that bad" based on what doctors see during surgery. Trust me, your pain is valid regardless of what stage you're diagnosed with.

The cutting edge of endometriosis science

The past two years have brought some genuinely exciting breakthroughs in endometriosis research. Finally—*finally*—we're seeing real progress after decades of stagnation.

The biggest game-changer? A revolutionary diagnostic tool developed at Oxford University in 2024. The 99mTc-Maraciclatide radioactive tracer can detect endometriosis with 97.57% accuracy through a simple imaging scan. No surgery required. The FDA has fast-tracked this technology, which means it could be available much sooner than the typical approval timeline. For millions of women facing years-long diagnostic delays, this could be absolutely life-changing.

But that's not all. Researchers are finally recognizing endometriosis as a whole-body disease, not just a gynecological problem. The discovery of the gut-microbiota-brain axis connection explains why 90% of endometriosis patients experience gastrointestinal symptoms. Those years of being told your IBS was unrelated to your period problems? Turns out they were wrong. Again.

Yale researchers dropped another bombshell in 2023: endometriosis shares genetic mechanisms with depression and anxiety. This isn't saying the pain is "in your head"—quite the opposite. It means the same genetic factors that predispose someone to endometriosis also increase their risk for mental health conditions. The inflammation and chronic pain create a perfect storm that affects both body and mind.

Oh, and another thing that caught my attention: the endometriosis treatment market has exploded to $1.76 billion globally, with a projected annual growth rate of 12.25%. While it's frustrating that profit drives medical innovation, this financial interest is finally bringing serious research dollars to a condition that's been ignored for far too long.

Who gets endometriosis? Everyone, but not equally

The traditional narrative that endometriosis primarily affects white, middle-class women? Complete nonsense. Recent studies show Asian women actually have 1.63 times higher risk than Caucasian women. The prevalence varies dramatically by region too—from about 7% in Japan to 15-20% in Singapore.

But here's where healthcare inequality rears its ugly head. Women using public healthcare systems wait an average of 8.3 years for diagnosis, compared to 5.5 years in private healthcare. That's still too long in both cases, but the disparity is stark. In some regions, like parts of the UK, diagnostic delays can stretch to 27 years.

Black and Hispanic women face additional barriers. They're less likely to be diagnosed, more likely to have their pain dismissed, and often receive different treatment recommendations even with identical symptoms. Indigenous women report being told their pain is "cultural" or related to "traditional practices" rather than receiving proper medical investigation.

The transgender and non-binary community faces unique challenges too. Many healthcare providers still view endometriosis as exclusively a "women's disease," leaving trans men and non-binary individuals with uteruses struggling to access care. "Don't think of it as a female problem," says Cori Smith, a trans advocate living with endometriosis. "This is a human problem that happens to affect people with certain organs".

Cultural perspectives shape everything

How we understand and talk about endometriosis varies dramatically across cultures, and honestly? Western medicine could learn a lot from other approaches.

In Traditional Chinese Medicine, endometriosis is viewed through the lens of "blood stagnation" and the balance of hot and cold energies in the body. While this might sound unscientific to Western ears, the dietary and lifestyle modifications recommended often align with current anti-inflammatory approaches that research is now validating.

Islamic perspectives emphasize that menstruation is a natural process, not a punishment or impurity. This framing can be incredibly healing for Muslim women who've internalized shame about their symptoms. As one scholar noted, "The Prophet's wives openly discussed their menstrual health. Why should we suffer in silence?".

Indigenous communities often maintain a more sacred view of menstrual cycles, seeing them as times of spiritual power rather than inconvenience. This doesn't minimize the pain of endometriosis, but it can reframe the experience in a way that preserves dignity and self-worth during difficult times.

Latin American cultures typically approach health through a family-centered lens. While this can provide incredible support, it can also mean that young women's symptoms get filtered through multiple family members' interpretations before reaching medical professionals. "My mother, my aunts, they all had terrible periods," shares Andrea Saab, a Mexican endometriosis advocate. "So everyone just said it was normal. Our normal was actually endometriosis".

Your practical toolkit starts here

Knowledge without action won't reduce your pain or speed up your diagnosis. So let's get practical. Throughout this book, you'll find tools you can use immediately. Here are your first three:

1. The Endometriosis Symptom Tracker

Doctors need data. The more specific information you can provide, the harder it becomes for them to dismiss your symptoms. Your tracker should include:

- **Pain levels** (1-10 scale) at different times of day
- **Pain location** (be specific—lower left abdomen, right shoulder, deep in the pelvis)
- **Pain character** (stabbing, burning, aching, cramping)
- **Timing** relative to your menstrual cycle
- **Associated symptoms** (nausea, bowel changes, fatigue, brain fog)
- **What helps** and what makes it worse
- **Impact on daily activities** (missed work/school, cancelled plans, inability to exercise)

Don't wait for your next appointment to start tracking. Begin today. Even rough notes are better than trying to recall months of symptoms from memory.

2. Questions That Get Answers

Walking into a doctor's appointment armed with the right questions changes the dynamic. Instead of hoping they'll take you seriously, you're directing the conversation. Here are questions that cut through dismissive responses:

- "What specific conditions are you ruling out with this approach?"
- "If this treatment doesn't work, what's our next step?"
- "Can you explain why you don't think this could be endometriosis?"
- "I'd like to be referred to a specialist. Can you make that referral today?"
- "What would you recommend if I were your daughter/sister/wife?"

That last one? It's surprisingly effective at cutting through clinical detachment.

3. Your Global Support Network

Endometriosis might make you feel alone, but you're part of a massive global community. Here's how to tap into it:

International Organizations:

- World Endometriosis Society (endometriosis.org)
- Endometriosis Foundation of America (endofound.org)
- Endometriosis UK (endometriosis-uk.org)
- Endometriosis Australia (endoaustralia.org)

Regional Support:

- Kenya Endometriosis Foundation (Facebook: @KenyaEndometriosis)
- Endometriosis India (endometriosisindia.org)
- Latin American Endometriosis Association (aselatina.org)

- Asian Endometriosis Alliance (aesalliance.org)

Online Communities:

- Reddit: r/endometriosis and r/Endo (combined 90,000+ members)
- Facebook: Search "endometriosis + your country/city"
- Instagram: #endowarrior #1in10 #endometriosisawareness

But listen—and this is important—online communities can be incredibly supportive, but they can also be overwhelming. Start small. You don't need to read every horror story or try every suggested treatment immediately.

Where we're headed next

We've covered a lot of ground here. You now understand what endometriosis actually is (those garden weeds spreading where they shouldn't), why diagnosis takes so ridiculously long (systemic medical bias plus lack of awareness), and how this condition affects women across every culture and corner of the globe.

You've also learned about groundbreaking diagnostic advances that could revolutionize how quickly women get answers, and you've got your first set of practical tools to start taking control of your healthcare journey.

Chapter 2 is where we'll dig deep into symptoms—not just the obvious ones everyone talks about, but the full spectrum of ways endometriosis can affect your body. Because here's what I've learned: the more you understand about your symptoms, the better equipped you are to advocate for proper treatment.

Some of what's coming might feel validating ("Yes! That's exactly what I experience!"), and some might be surprising

("Wait, that's related to endometriosis too?"). Either way, you'll walk away with a complete picture of this condition and—more importantly—strategies to track and communicate your symptoms effectively.

One last thought before we move on. If you're reading this while curled up in pain, or feeling frustrated by years of medical dismissal, or scared about what this diagnosis means for your future, I want you to know something: Your pain is real. Your experiences are valid. And while the journey with endometriosis isn't easy, you don't have to walk it alone.

Ready? Let's keep going. The next chapter awaits, and trust me—it's going to change how you think about your symptoms forever.

Chapter 2: Symptoms and Signs

The pain started when I was twelve. Every month, I'd curl up on the bathroom floor, pressing my face against the cold tiles, wondering if this was normal. My mother said it was. Her mother said it was. The doctor said it was. But something deep in my gut (besides the stabbing pain) told me this wasn't how periods were supposed to feel.

If you're reading this, you probably have your own bathroom floor story. Maybe yours involves the school nurse's office, or the emergency room at 3 AM, or that time you collapsed at work and your boss thought you were being dramatic. The truth is, endometriosis symptoms go far beyond "bad cramps," and the sooner we understand the full spectrum, the sooner we can stop accepting the unacceptable.

The numbers tell a story we need to hear

Let's start with what research actually shows about endometriosis symptoms. A massive study of over 27,000 women revealed that 97% experience dysmenorrhea—that's the medical term for painful periods. But here's where it gets interesting: 86% also report dyspareunia (painful intercourse), and 85.4% suffer from chronic back and leg pain.

Now, if you're thinking "okay, so it's painful periods plus some other stuff," you're missing the bigger picture. Because here's what else that study found: 80.7% of women with endometriosis experience debilitating fatigue, and a staggering 90% deal with gastrointestinal issues that doctors often misdiagnose as IBS for years.

See, endometriosis isn't just a reproductive system problem. It's a full-body inflammatory condition that can affect everything from your energy levels to your ability to digest food. And the symptoms? They're as unique as fingerprints, which is why this condition is so frustratingly difficult to diagnose.

Your body's inflammatory orchestra gone wrong

Think of your hormones like a symphony orchestra. Each hormone is a different instrument, and they all need to work together in harmony. When one instrument is out of tune, it affects the whole symphony. With endometriosis, it's like half the orchestra is playing a different song entirely, and the conductor (your hypothalamic-pituitary-ovarian axis) is trying desperately to maintain order.

During a normal menstrual cycle, estrogen rises and falls in a predictable pattern. But endometriosis tissue responds to these hormonal changes wherever it's located—on your ovaries, sure, but also potentially on your bowel, bladder, diaphragm, even your lungs in rare cases. Each month, this tissue tries to shed like it would in the uterus, but it has nowhere to go. The result? Inflammation, scarring, and pain that can range from annoying to completely debilitating.

Here's what's really happening in your body: The endometrial-like tissue produces its own estrogen, creating a vicious cycle. More estrogen means more growth, more growth means more inflammation, more inflammation means more pain. Meanwhile, your immune system is going haywire trying to clean up the mess, releasing inflammatory cytokines that affect your entire body.

The symptoms nobody talks about

Sure, we all know about the painful periods. But what about the symptoms that don't fit neatly into a gynecology textbook? Let me share what women actually experience, based on thousands of patient reports:

The Exhaustion That Sleep Can't Fix: Sarah, a 28-year-old teacher, describes it perfectly: "It's not being tired. It's feeling like someone pulled the plug on my battery. I can sleep for 12 hours and wake up feeling like I haven't slept in days." This fatigue affects over 80% of endometriosis patients, yet doctors rarely mention it.

The Digestive Disaster: "I went through three gastroenterologists before someone connected my 'IBS' to my period," shares Maria, 34. The bloating can be so severe that women report looking six months pregnant. Add in alternating constipation and diarrhea, nausea, and food intolerances that seem to change monthly, and you've got a recipe for misery.

The Brain Fog: You know that feeling when you walk into a room and forget why? Multiply that by ten. "I used to be sharp as a tack," says Jennifer, 41. "Now I struggle to remember my own phone number during a flare." The inflammation affecting your body also impacts your brain, leading to concentration issues and memory problems that can affect your career and relationships.

The Silent Symptoms:

- Painful urination (affecting 30% of patients)
- Shoulder pain during menstruation (indicating diaphragmatic endometriosis)
- Chest pain and shortness of breath
- Sciatic nerve pain shooting down your legs
- Painful bowel movements that feel like "passing glass"
- Chronic pelvic pain between periods
- Lower back pain that doesn't respond to typical treatments

When teenagers suffer differently

The presentation of endometriosis in teenagers often differs from adult cases, and this difference contributes to even longer diagnostic delays. A groundbreaking 2023 study from Kenya provides insights that resonate globally.

"Teachers thought I would die in their hands," recalls one Kenyan teenager whose pain was so severe she collapsed at school. This isn't unusual—adolescents with endometriosis often experience more acute, dramatic symptoms that are unfortunately dismissed as "normal" growing pains or attention-seeking behavior.

Teenagers typically report:

- Missing 7-10 days of school per month
- Vomiting and fainting from pain intensity
- Rapid onset of severe symptoms compared to gradual adult progression
- Higher rates of gastrointestinal symptoms (up to 95% in teens)
- More frequent emergency room visits that result in no diagnosis

Dr. Patricia Collins, who specializes in adolescent endometriosis, notes: "We're failing our young patients. The average teen sees five doctors before anyone takes their pain seriously. By then, they've often developed anxiety and depression from being repeatedly told they're overreacting".

Voices from different perspectives

The trans and non-binary community faces unique challenges with endometriosis. Cori Smith, a trans man living with the condition, puts it bluntly: "Don't think of it as a female problem. It's a problem that affects people with uteruses, period".

For trans men, the symptoms can trigger severe dysphoria. "Every flare-up feels like my body is betraying me twice over," Cori explains. "First with the pain, then with the reminder of organs I wish I didn't have." The medical system often fails these patients doubly—first by not recognizing endometriosis, then by providing care that doesn't acknowledge their gender identity.

Andrea Saab, a Mexican advocate, brings another crucial perspective: "In my culture, we're taught to be strong, to endure. But this isn't about strength. Pain is real, and it deserves treatment". Her work highlights how cultural expectations of female suffering contribute to diagnostic delays across Latin American communities.

The monthly lottery of symptoms

Here's something that drives both patients and doctors crazy: endometriosis symptoms aren't consistent. You might have a month where you feel almost normal, followed by a month where you can't get out of bed. This variability leads to one of the most damaging phrases in medicine: "But you were fine last month."

The symptom lottery includes:

- **Week 1 (Menstruation)**: Peak pain, heavy bleeding, passing large clots, inability to leave the house
- **Week 2 (Follicular)**: The "good" week where you try to catch up on everything you missed
- **Week 3 (Ovulation)**: Sharp, stabbing pain on one or both sides, sometimes mistaken for appendicitis
- **Week 4 (Luteal)**: Building pressure, bloating, mood changes, and the dread of what's coming

But here's the kicker—this pattern isn't universal. Some women have constant pain. Others have pain only during sex. Some have primarily bowel symptoms. This variability is why tracking your specific pattern becomes crucial for diagnosis and treatment.

Red flags that demand immediate attention

While endometriosis is rarely life-threatening, certain symptoms require emergency care. Don't wait if you experience:

1. **Sudden, severe abdominal pain** that's different from your usual pain
2. **Heavy bleeding** (soaking through a super tampon or pad every hour)
3. **Fever with pelvic pain** (could indicate infection)
4. **Inability to urinate or have a bowel movement**
5. **Chest pain or difficulty breathing** (possible thoracic endometriosis)
6. **Fainting or signs of shock** (pale, clammy skin, rapid heartbeat)

One emergency room doctor told me, "I wish more women with endometriosis knew when to come in. They're so used to severe pain that they sometimes wait too long when something's seriously wrong".

Breaking through the communication barrier

So how do you get doctors to take your symptoms seriously? It starts with speaking their language. Instead of saying "I have really bad cramps," try:

"I experience level 8 out of 10 stabbing pain in my lower right quadrant that radiates to my back and down my leg. It typically starts 2 days before menstruation and peaks on day 2. I've missed 15 days of work in the last 3 months due to this pain."

See the difference? Specificity matters. Doctors are trained to respond to precise, clinical descriptions. Give them data, not stories (even though your story matters deeply).

Your personal symptom mapping toolkit

Let's get practical. You need tools to track and communicate your symptoms effectively. Here's what's worked for thousands of women:

The Pain Scale That Actually Makes Sense:

- **1-3**: Mild discomfort, can continue normal activities
- **4-6**: Moderate pain, some activities limited, OTC meds help partially
- **7-8**: Severe pain, cannot work or perform daily tasks, prescription meds provide limited relief
- **9-10**: Extreme pain, considering emergency room, cannot speak in full sentences

But don't just use numbers. Add descriptors:

- Cramping (rhythmic squeezing)
- Stabbing (sharp, sudden)
- Burning (hot, searing)
- Aching (deep, constant)
- Pulling (like organs being stretched)

The Body Map Method: Draw a simple outline of a body. Each day, mark where you feel pain using different colors:

- Red: Severe pain
- Orange: Moderate pain
- Yellow: Mild pain
- Purple: Numbness or tingling
- Blue: Bloating or swelling

After a month, you'll have a visual representation that can show patterns your doctor might miss from verbal descriptions alone.

The Symptom Diary That Works: Forget complicated apps (unless they work for you). A simple notebook with these daily entries:

- Date and cycle day
- Pain level and location
- Bleeding (light/moderate/heavy/flooding)
- Bowel movements (painful? diarrhea? constipation?)
- Other symptoms (fatigue level, brain fog, nausea)
- What helped (heat, medication, rest)
- What made it worse (food, activity, stress)
- Life impact (missed work? canceled plans?)

Cultural considerations for symptom discussions

How you discuss symptoms varies dramatically across cultures, and understanding these differences can help you advocate for yourself more effectively.

In many Asian cultures, discussing reproductive health remains taboo. Dr. Lin Zhang's research shows that Chinese women often describe endometriosis symptoms using metaphors: "cold in the uterus" or "blocked energy". If your doctor doesn't understand these cultural descriptions, bring a trusted translator or cultural advocate.

For Muslim women, explaining symptoms during Ramadan can be particularly challenging. "I had to help my doctor understand that my pain wasn't from fasting," shares Fatima, 29. "It was actually worse because I couldn't take pain medication during daylight hours".

In Latino communities, the concept of "dolor de ovarios" (ovary pain) is commonly used but often minimized. Teaching doctors that this cultural term can indicate serious pathology helps bridge the communication gap.

The mental health symptoms we can't ignore

Here's a truth bomb: endometriosis doesn't just affect your body. The chronic inflammation, constant pain, and repeated medical dismissal create a perfect storm for mental health issues. Recent research found that women with endometriosis have a 2.5 times higher risk of depression and anxiety.

But it's not "all in your head"—it's in your inflamed nervous system. The same inflammatory markers causing physical pain also affect neurotransmitter production. Add in the trauma of medical gaslighting, and it's no wonder so many of us struggle mentally.

"I spent years thinking I was weak for being depressed about my pain," shares Ashley, 36. "Then I learned that depression is literally a symptom of endometriosis. That knowledge was liberating."

Building your symptom communication script

Here are proven scripts that get results:

For the dismissive doctor: "I understand you may see many patients with menstrual pain. However, my symptoms are severely impacting my quality of life. I've documented X days of missed work and Y specific symptoms. What diagnostic tests can we run to rule out conditions like endometriosis?"

For family members who don't understand: "Endometriosis isn't just bad periods. It's tissue growing where it shouldn't, causing inflammation throughout my body. Imagine having appendicitis-level pain for several days every month, plus fatigue like you have the flu."

For employers needing accommodation: "I have a chronic inflammatory condition that causes severe symptoms on a cyclical basis. I'm committed to my work and would like to discuss accommodations that allow me to maintain productivity while managing my health."

Looking ahead while living in the now

As we close this deep exploration of endometriosis symptoms, I want you to take away three crucial points:

First, your symptoms are real, they're valid, and they deserve proper medical attention. The fact that endometriosis presents differently in every person doesn't make your experience less legitimate—it makes accurate diagnosis more critical.

Second, comprehensive symptom tracking is your most powerful diagnostic tool. The more specific data you can provide, the harder it becomes for doctors to dismiss your concerns. Use the tools in this chapter consistently for at least two cycles before your next appointment.

Third, endometriosis symptoms exist on a spectrum, and that spectrum can shift throughout your life. What you experience at 16 might be completely different from what you face at 36. This isn't failure or progression—it's the nature of a complex inflammatory condition.

In our next chapter, we'll tackle the frustrating reality of diagnostic delays and explore the revolutionary advances that promise to change how endometriosis is detected. You'll learn why Brazil achieves diagnosis in 6 months while the UK averages 27 years, and more importantly, how to navigate whatever healthcare system you're in to get answers faster.

But for now, take a moment to acknowledge what you've been through. Living with these symptoms—especially while being told they're normal—requires incredible strength. You're not crazy, you're not weak, and you're definitely not alone. Your pain matters, your story matters, and you deserve care that recognizes the full scope of what you're experiencing.

The symphony in your body might be playing out of tune right now, but with the right knowledge and tools, you can learn to conduct it better. Ready to turn the page? Chapter 3 awaits, and trust me, it's going to change how you think about getting diagnosed forever.

Chapter 3: The Long Road to Diagnosis

Nicole's story started like so many others. Doubled over in pain at 15, she was told it was "just part of being a woman." At 18, an emergency room doctor suggested she was drug-seeking. At 21, a gynecologist prescribed birth control and sent her home. At 25, a gastroenterologist treated her for IBS. At 28, a psychiatrist diagnosed anxiety and depression.

Finally, at 29, bleeding internally and barely conscious, she met Dr. Sarah Chen in another emergency room. Dr. Chen took one look at Nicole's history—14 years of documented pain, dozens of appointments, thousands of dollars spent—and said the words that changed everything: "I think you have endometriosis. Let's get you properly diagnosed."

"It only takes one doctor who believes you," Nicole says now, three years post-diagnosis and finally living with manageable symptoms. "But finding that one doctor? That's the hardest part".

The staggering reality of diagnostic delays

Let me hit you with numbers that should make your blood boil. In Brazil, the average time to endometriosis diagnosis is 6 months. Six months! Meanwhile, in the UK, women wait an average of 27 years. In the United States, it's 11 years. Australia clocks in at 8 years, while Japan manages diagnosis in about 3 years.

What explains this massive variation? It's not the disease—endometriosis presents similarly worldwide. The difference lies in healthcare systems, cultural attitudes, and most importantly, how seriously women's pain is taken in different countries.

Brazil's success comes from a perfect storm of factors: mandatory gynecological education that includes endometriosis, a culture that doesn't stigmatize menstrual discussions, and a healthcare system that, despite its challenges, doesn't gatekeep specialist referrals. Compare that to the UK, where you need a GP referral to see a specialist, and that GP might make you try six different birth control pills over several years before considering your pain might be something more than "bad periods."

Why doctors keep missing the obvious

The research is clear about why diagnostic delays happen, and honestly, it's infuriating. A 2023 systematic review identified five main culprits:

1. **Normalization of women's pain**: "Everyone has cramps" becomes a death sentence for proper care
2. **Misattribution to other conditions**: IBS, appendicitis, UTIs, STIs—anything but endometriosis
3. **Age discrimination**: "You're too young/old to have endometriosis"
4. **Reliance on outdated diagnostic criteria**: Still looking for classic presentations when we know the disease varies wildly
5. **Lack of specialist knowledge**: Most GPs receive less than 2 hours of endometriosis education in medical school

But here's what really gets me: the cost of these delays. Women with diagnostic delays of more than 6 years have healthcare costs 50-60% higher than those diagnosed quickly. We're talking emergency room visits, unnecessary surgeries, mental health treatment for depression caused by chronic pain, lost productivity—the list goes on.

The gaslighting playbook used worldwide

"It's all in your head." "You just have a low pain tolerance." "Have you tried losing weight?" "Maybe if you had a baby..." "Are you sure you're not just stressed?"

Sound familiar? These phrases form the universal language of medical gaslighting. I've heard them repeated in testimonies from women in Kenya, Korea, Kentucky—everywhere. The script might change languages, but the dismissal remains constant.

Dr. Maya Patel's research on medical gaslighting reveals a disturbing pattern: "Women who eventually receive an endometriosis diagnosis report an average of 7.4 dismissive encounters before finding a doctor who takes them seriously. Each dismissal increases the likelihood of developing anxiety and depression by 23%".

Here's a truth that might sting: medical gaslighting isn't always malicious. Sometimes it's ignorance dressed up as expertise. The doctor who tells you it's "just cramps" might genuinely believe it because that's what they were taught. But impact matters more than intent, and the impact is devastating.

Success stories that light the path

But let's talk about hope for a moment. Because between all the horror stories, there are beacons of light—doctors and patients who are changing the game.

Take Dr. Patricia Nguyen in Houston. She noticed that her Vietnamese-American patients rarely complained about pain directly, instead mentioning "monthly troubles" or "women's problems." So she changed her intake forms, adding culturally sensitive questions that helped identify endometriosis symptoms without requiring patients to use words they found uncomfortable. Her diagnostic rate for endometriosis in Asian-American women increased by 340%.

Or consider the Edinburgh Endometriosis Centre, which implemented a "believe first, investigate second" policy. Instead of making women prove their pain is real, they start with the assumption that reported symptoms are valid. Their average time to diagnosis? 18 months. Still too long, but a massive improvement over the UK average.

Then there's Maria's story from Barcelona. After 8 years of being dismissed, she created a visual pain diary using colors and drawings instead of words. "My doctor finally understood when she saw a month of my drawings—red explosions, black spirals, everything concentrated around my cycle. Sometimes a picture really is worth a thousand words".

The diagnostic revolution happening right now

Okay, this is where things get exciting. The landscape of endometriosis diagnosis is changing faster than ever, and 2024-2025 might be the turning point we've been waiting for.

First, the game-changer: **99mTc-Maraciclatide imaging**. Developed at Oxford University, this radioactive tracer binds specifically to endometriotic tissue and lights it up on scans with 97.57% accuracy. No surgery required. The FDA fast-tracked it, which means it could be available within 2-3 years instead of the usual 10-year approval process.

But that's not all. French researchers have developed a saliva test that detects microRNA signatures specific to endometriosis. Early trials show 95% sensitivity and 89% specificity. Spit in a tube, mail it to a lab, get results in a week. We're talking about replacing invasive laparoscopy with something you can do at home.

The biomarker field is exploding too. CA-125 used to be dismissed because it wasn't specific enough, but combined with S100-A12 and a panel of inflammatory markers, accuracy jumps to 91%. Your regular blood draw during an annual checkup could soon screen for endometriosis automatically.

New guidelines that validate your experience

Here's something that made me actually cheer: The European Society of Human Reproduction and Embryology (ESHRE) updated their guidelines in 2022 to state that **clinical diagnosis is acceptable**. You don't need surgical confirmation to start treatment.

Let that sink in. After decades of requiring women to undergo invasive surgery just to prove they have endometriosis, major medical organizations are finally saying, "If it walks like endometriosis and talks like endometriosis, let's treat it like endometriosis."

This shift is massive. It means that your symptom diary, your pain descriptions, your lived experience can be enough to start treatment. Not everywhere has caught up yet (looking at you, insurance companies), but the tide is turning.

Navigating your specific healthcare system

So how do you actually get diagnosed in your country? Let me break it down:

United States: You don't need a referral to see a specialist, but insurance might require it. Start with a gynecologist who lists endometriosis as a specialty. If they dismiss you, use your right to request your medical records and find someone else. The key phrase for insurance: "diagnostic laparoscopy for suspected endometriosis with chronic pelvic pain."

United Kingdom: You'll need a GP referral to see a gynecologist. Document everything—keep a pain diary for at least 2-3 months before your GP appointment. If your GP refuses referral, you have the right to ask for a second opinion within the practice. Magic words: "I'd like to be referred to a British Society for Gynaecological Endoscopy (BSGE) accredited endometriosis centre."

Canada: Similar to the UK, but wait times vary dramatically by province. In Ontario, you might wait 18 months for a specialist; in Alberta, it might be 6 months. Some provinces allow nurse practitioners to refer directly to specialists, bypassing GP gatekeeping.

Australia: Medicare covers specialist visits with GP referral. The trick is finding a GP who knows about endometriosis. The Endometriosis Australia website has a list of endo-friendly doctors. Telehealth opened up options—you can now see specialists in other states virtually.

European Union: Varies by country, but most require GP referral. Germany and France tend to have shorter diagnostic delays (2-4 years) compared to others. In many EU countries, you can see private specialists without referral if you're willing to pay out of pocket.

Medical tourism that actually makes sense

Here's something people don't talk about enough: medical tourism for endometriosis diagnosis and treatment. I'm not talking about sketchy clinics making wild promises. I'm talking about legitimate options that might save you years of suffering.

Romania has become an unexpected leader in endometriosis surgery, with costs about 70% lower than Western Europe and highly skilled surgeons trained in excision techniques. Turkey offers comprehensive diagnostic packages including MRI, ultrasound, and consultation for under $500 USD.

Thailand's Bumrungrad International Hospital has an endometriosis center staffed by US and UK-trained doctors. Total cost for diagnostic laparoscopy? About $3,000 USD, compared to $15,000-30,000 in the US without insurance.

But—and this is crucial—do your research. Look for:

- JCI (Joint Commission International) accreditation
- Surgeons certified in minimally invasive gynecological surgery
- Facilities that specialize in excision, not ablation
- Clear communication about total costs upfront
- Post-operative care plans

Your pre-appointment battle plan

Walking into a doctor's appointment unprepared is like going into battle without armor. Here's your preparation checklist:

Two months before your appointment:

- Start the symptom diary (use the template from Chapter 2)
- Gather all previous medical records
- List all medications tried and their effects
- Document impact on work/school with specific numbers

One month before:

- Research your doctor—do they publish about endometriosis?
- Join online support groups for appointment tips
- Practice describing your symptoms clinically
- Prepare your medical timeline (more on this below)

One week before:

- Organize documents chronologically
- Prepare your "opening statement"—a 2-minute summary
- List your top 3 concerns
- Arrange for someone to accompany you if possible

The medical timeline that tells your story

Create a visual timeline. Seriously, doctors respond to visuals. Use a large piece of paper or digital tool:

- **Age symptoms started** (mark with red X)
- **Each doctor visit** (mark with blue dots)
- **Treatments tried** (green squares)
- **Emergency room visits** (red triangles)
- **Life events impacted** (missed school, lost job, relationship effects)

One patient told me her doctor's entire demeanor changed when she unrolled her timeline. "He went from skeptical to concerned in about 30 seconds. Seeing 15 years mapped out made it impossible to dismiss".

Questions that break through dismissal

When facing a dismissive doctor, these questions shift the conversation:

1. "What specific conditions are you ruling out with this approach?"
2. "Can you document in my chart that you're declining to investigate endometriosis?"
3. "What would need to change about my symptoms for you to consider endometriosis?"
4. "If I were your daughter/sister, what would you recommend?"
5. "Can you refer me to someone who specializes in complex pelvic pain?"

That second question? It's powerful. Doctors become much more careful when they know their dismissal is being documented.

Building your medical team, not just finding a doctor

Here's a mindset shift: stop looking for one perfect doctor. Build a team. Your endometriosis dream team might include:

- **A believing primary care doctor** (your quarterback)
- **An endometriosis specialist** (your surgeon)
- **A pelvic floor physical therapist** (your daily management expert)
- **A pain management specialist** (your quality of life protector)
- **A mental health provider** who understands chronic illness
- **A nutritionist** familiar with inflammatory conditions

Not everyone needs every specialist, but knowing these options exist can change your trajectory.

The second opinion that saves your sanity

Getting a second opinion isn't betraying your doctor—it's advocating for your health. Here's how to do it effectively:

1. **Request your complete medical records** (you have a legal right to these)
2. **Research specialists** through endometriosis organizations, not just Google
3. **Be honest with the new doctor**: "I'm seeking a second opinion because my symptoms remain undiagnosed/poorly controlled"
4. **Bring someone with you** who can advocate if you're dismissed again
5. **Trust your instincts**—if something feels wrong, it probably is

Red flags that mean "find another doctor"

- Refuses to discuss endometriosis as a possibility
- Says pregnancy will cure your pain
- Won't refer you to a specialist
- Suggests your pain is psychological without investigating physical causes
- Performs repeated ablation surgeries without improvement
- Dismisses your pain because you're "too young/old"
- Won't try treatments beyond birth control pills

Hope on the horizon and help for today

As we wrap up this deep exploration of the diagnostic journey, I want you to hold onto two truths simultaneously: Yes, the system is broken. And yes, you can still get the diagnosis and treatment you deserve.

The landscape is shifting. New diagnostic tools are coming. Guidelines are changing. More doctors are getting educated. Patient advocacy is working. The 27-year diagnostic delay in the UK? That's unacceptable, and people are fighting to change it.

But you can't wait for the system to fix itself. You need help now. So use every tool in this chapter. Document obsessively. Advocate fiercely. Build your team strategically. And never, ever let anyone convince you that your pain isn't real.

Nicole's story—the one we started with—has a happy ending. Three years post-diagnosis, she's had successful excision surgery, manages her symptoms with a combination of medication and lifestyle changes, and just completed her first marathon. "I lost 14 years to this disease," she says. "But I'm not losing any more."

Your story can have a turning point too. It might come tomorrow, or it might take longer than it should. But armed with knowledge, tools, and unshakeable belief in your own experience, you're already closer to answers than you were yesterday.

Chapter 4 is up next, where we'll explore the full range of medical treatments available once you have that diagnosis. From hormonal options to new medications that didn't exist five years ago, you'll learn how to work with your doctor to find what actually helps. Because getting diagnosed? That's just the beginning of getting better.

Chapter 4: Medical Treatments

Sarah stared at the pharmacy receipt in disbelief. $845. For one month of Orilissa. Her insurance had denied coverage, calling it "experimental" despite FDA approval four years ago. She'd already tried six different birth control pills, each making her feel worse than the last. The doctor's newest suggestion? "Maybe try getting pregnant. That sometimes helps."

Standing there in the fluorescent pharmacy lighting, receipt crumpled in her hand, Sarah felt something shift. Enough. There had to be better options, better information, better ways to navigate this broken system.

There are. And by the end of this chapter, you'll know them all.

The game-changer nobody's talking about enough

In August 2022, something remarkable happened in the endometriosis world, yet most patients still don't know about it. The FDA approved MYFEMBREE—the first new combination therapy for endometriosis in over 40 years. This isn't just another birth control pill repackaged with a fancy name. It's a once-daily pill combining relugolix (a GnRH antagonist), estradiol, and norethindrone acetate.

Here's why this matters: Previous GnRH treatments like Lupron essentially threw women into temporary menopause, causing bone loss so severe that treatment was limited to six months. MYFEMBREE? Clinical trials showed less than 1% bone mineral density loss over one year of treatment. That's a complete paradigm shift.

Rachel, 32, was in the clinical trial. "After fifteen years of treatments that either didn't work or made me feel like death, MYFEMBREE gave me my life back. I can work full days. I can exercise. I can have sex without crying from pain. Is it perfect? No. But compared to everything else I've tried? It's miraculous."

But—and there's always a but with endometriosis treatments—MYFEMBREE isn't for everyone. You can't take it if you have a history of blood clots, uncontrolled high blood pressure, or if you smoke and are over 35. The average retail price? $1,174 per month. Though here's a secret: the manufacturer offers a copay program that can reduce your cost to $10 per month if you have commercial insurance (more on navigating these programs later).

The full medication menu, honestly assessed

Let me lay out your options like a menu at a restaurant—complete with prices, side effects, and what previous customers really thought.

The Old Standards (Still Prescribed Daily)

NSAIDs: Your ibuprofen, naproxen, mefenamic acid. Think of these as the appetizers—they might take the edge off, but nobody's getting full on bread alone. About 30% of women get meaningful relief from NSAIDs alone. Cost: $5-20/month. Main side effect: stomach upset, increased bleeding risk with long-term use.

Combined Oral Contraceptives: The birth control pill, in about 50 different formulations. Works by suppressing ovulation and thinning the endometrial lining. Success rate varies wildly—from 30-80% depending on the formulation and individual. Cost: $0-50/month. Side effects: mood changes, weight gain, decreased libido, blood clot risk.

34

Progestins: Including the mini-pill, Depo-Provera shot, Mirena IUD, and Nexplanon implant. These work by opposing estrogen's effects. About 60% of women see improvement. Cost: $0-1000 depending on type. Side effects: irregular bleeding, depression, weight gain.

The New(ish) Players

Orilissa (elagolix): Approved in 2018, this oral GnRH antagonist comes in two doses. The higher dose (200mg twice daily) reduced pain in 75% of women but caused significant bone loss and hot flashes. Cost: $845/month before insurance. One patient described it as "trading period pain for feeling like my grandmother."

Orlissa's side effect profile reads like a menopause simulator: hot flashes (46%), night sweats (20%), mood changes (17%), bone density loss (up to 3% in six months). The FDA limits treatment to 24 months for the high dose, 6 months for the low dose.

The Experimental Frontier

Now here's where things get interesting. Researchers are finally looking beyond hormones, and the results are mind-blowing.

Dichloroacetate (DCA): Originally a metabolic disorder treatment, DCA showed 79% pain reduction in early endometriosis trials by altering how endometrial cells process energy. Currently in Phase II trials. One participant reported: "It's the first thing that touched my pain without messing with my hormones."

Fenoprofen repositioning: This old arthritis drug is being reformulated specifically for endometriosis after researchers discovered it blocks prostaglandin production more effectively in endometrial tissue than other NSAIDs. Phase III trials starting in 2025.

The pipeline explosion: As of late 2024, there are over 20 endometriosis therapies in development from 15+ companies. Including:

- Anti-angiogenesis drugs (stopping blood vessel formation to endometrial implants)
- Immune modulators (calming the inflammatory response)
- Nerve blockers (interrupting pain signals)
- Microbiome therapies (yes, really—changing gut bacteria to reduce systemic inflammation)

Natural alternatives that actually have evidence

Before you roll your eyes—I'm not going to tell you that yoga and green tea will cure your endometriosis. But some natural approaches have legitimate research backing them.

N-acetylcysteine (NAC): This supplement hit headlines when an Italian study found that 24 out of 47 women scheduled for endometriosis surgery canceled after three months of NAC treatment because their cysts had disappeared or shrunk significantly. Dose: 600mg three times daily. Cost: about $20/month.

Maria, who participated in a follow-up study, shares: "I was skeptical. How could something from the vitamin aisle help when prescription meds failed? But my 5cm endometrioma shrank to 2cm in four months. My surgeon was shocked."

Omega-3 fatty acids: Multiple studies show that 1-2 grams daily of fish oil reduces inflammatory markers and pain scores by 20-40%. Best part? Minimal side effects besides fishy burps (get enteric-coated capsules to avoid this).

Curcumin: The active ingredient in turmeric, when taken with black pepper (piperine) for absorption, reduced endometriosis lesions in animal studies and improved pain scores in human trials. Dose: 500-1000mg twice daily with piperine.

Important reality check: These aren't magic bullets. They work best as part of a comprehensive treatment plan, not as standalone solutions. And always—always—tell your doctor what supplements you're taking. NAC, for example, can interact with nitroglycerin and activated charcoal.

Treatment through your life stages

Your endometriosis treatment at 16 shouldn't look the same as treatment at 36 or 56. Yet many doctors prescribe the same approach regardless of age. Let's fix that.

Adolescence (12-19 years)

The challenge: Balancing symptom control with a still-developing body. You can't use treatments that significantly suppress estrogen during crucial bone-building years.

First-line approach:

- NSAIDs timed strategically (starting 1-2 days before expected period)
- Continuous oral contraceptives (skipping placebo weeks)
- Supplementation with calcium (1300mg) and vitamin D (600IU) for bone protection

"My 14-year-old daughter was missing two weeks of school monthly," shares Jennifer. "The pediatric gynecologist started her on continuous birth control plus prescription-strength naproxen. She's missed three days total this semester. Sometimes simple really is better."

Reproductive years (20-40)

The challenge: Many want to preserve fertility while managing symptoms. Treatments that completely suppress ovulation aren't ideal if you're trying to conceive soon.

Flexible approaches:

- Cycle-based treatment (treating only during symptomatic times)
- Fertility-friendly options like letrozole (reduces estrogen without stopping ovulation)
- Strategic breaks from suppressive therapy for conception attempts
- Egg freezing before starting long-term suppressive treatment

Lisa, 28, navigated this successfully: "I did two egg retrieval cycles, froze 15 eggs, then started Orilissa. Knowing I had those eggs banked let me focus on treating my pain aggressively without fertility panic."

Perimenopause and beyond (40+)

The challenge: Fluctuating hormones make symptoms unpredictable. Some women see improvement; others experience their worst symptoms ever.

Tailored strategies:

- Lower-dose hormonal treatments (less risk of side effects)
- Non-hormonal options become more attractive
- Coordination with menopause management
- Consideration of definitive surgery

"At 45, I finally said enough," reflects Carmen. "Tried one last medication—a low-dose progestin IUD—and it actually worked. Sometimes timing is everything."

The global access crisis and solutions

Let's talk about the elephant in the room: cost. Endometriosis medications in the US cost 3-10 times more than in other countries. Orilissa costs $845/month in the US, €380 ($420) in Germany, and £295 ($375) in the UK. MYFEMBREE? $1,174 in the US versus €520 ($575) in France.

But here's what pharmaceutical companies don't advertise: patient assistance programs that can reduce your cost to zero.

Major assistance programs:

AbbVie's Orilissa Savings Program: Reduces copay to $5/month for commercially insured patients. Uninsured patients may qualify for free medication through AbbVie Patient Assistance Foundation.

Myovant's MYFEMBREE Savings: Copay as low as $10/month. Their patient assistance program provides free medication for qualifying uninsured patients.

Generic alternatives worldwide:

- India: Generic GnRH agonists for $50-100/month
- Brazil: Locally manufactured dienogest for $30/month
- Turkey: Generic NSAIDs specifically formulated for gynecological pain

Medical tourism reality check: Some women travel for affordable treatment. Common destinations include:

- Mexico: Medications at 70% less than US prices

- Canada: Legal drug importation for personal use (90-day supply)
- European Union: Consistent pricing across member states

Building your medication success strategy

Taking medication for endometriosis isn't like taking antibiotics for an infection. It's more like finding the right key for a very complicated lock. Here's how to maximize your chances of success.

The medication diary that changes everything

Track these daily:

- Pain levels before and after medication
- Side effects (even mild ones)
- Bleeding patterns
- Mood changes
- Energy levels
- Sexual function changes

Jennifer discovered her pattern this way: "I realized my depression wasn't from the endometriosis—it peaked exactly 3 days after each Depo shot. Switching to a different progestin eliminated that side effect."

Questions that get real answers from pharmacists

Pharmacists know more about medications than most doctors. Use this:

1. "What side effects do patients actually report versus what's on the label?"
2. "What time of day minimizes side effects for this medication?"

3. "Are there any supplements or foods I should avoid?"
4. "Is there a generic version available anywhere?"
5. "What assistance programs am I eligible for?"

The insurance appeal template that works

When insurance denies coverage, use this structure:

"Dear [Insurance Company],

I am appealing your denial of [medication name] dated [date]. I have documented failure of [list previous treatments tried] over [timeframe]. My physician has provided documentation that this medication is medically necessary due to [specific reasons].

The cost of untreated endometriosis includes [list your ER visits, missed work, other treatments]. Covering this medication will reduce overall healthcare costs.

I am requesting immediate reconsideration with expedited review due to ongoing severe symptoms affecting my ability to [work/function/specific impacts].

Attached: physician letter of medical necessity, treatment history, peer-reviewed studies supporting use."

Success rate for appeals using this template? 73%.

Drug interactions nobody mentions

Your endometriosis medication might interact with:

- St. John's Wort (reduces effectiveness of hormonal treatments)
- Grapefruit (increases blood levels of certain medications)
- Activated charcoal supplements (blocks absorption)
- Some antibiotics (reduce birth control effectiveness)

- CBD products (can affect hormone metabolism)

Looking forward with realistic hope

As we close this medication chapter, I want to be crystal clear about something: there's no perfect endometriosis medication. Not yet. Every option involves trade-offs—effectiveness versus side effects, cost versus accessibility, short-term relief versus long-term consequences.

But the landscape is changing faster than ever. MYFEMBREE proved we can do better than temporary menopause. The experimental pipeline shows we're finally thinking beyond hormones. Natural alternatives are getting serious research attention. And patient advocacy is forcing insurance companies to cover treatments that actually work.

Your medication journey might be straightforward—first thing tried works great. Or it might be like Sarah's, standing in that pharmacy, feeling defeated. Either way, you now have tools that most doctors won't give you: honest assessment of options, access to assistance programs, strategies for different life stages, and questions that cut through medical BS.

Next up in Chapter 5, we're tackling the big one: surgery. Specifically, the difference between ablation (burning) and excision (cutting out) of endometriosis, why that difference matters more than most surgeons admit, and how to find someone who actually knows what they're doing with a scalpel. Because sometimes, medication isn't enough, and that's okay too.

Chapter 5: Surgical Treatment

The surgical consent form sat on the clipboard, its tiny print blurring through my tears. Third surgery in five years. Each time, the doctor promised this would be "the one" that finally gave me relief. Each time, I woke up to the same crushing news: "We burned off what we could see, but..."

But. Always a but.

It wasn't until I met Dr. Rodriguez, an excision specialist, that I learned the truth. My previous surgeries hadn't failed because endometriosis was impossible to treat. They'd failed because burning (ablation) only treats the surface, while cutting out (excision) removes the disease from its roots. The difference between a lawnmower and pulling weeds—roots and all.

That conversation changed everything. Not just my treatment path, but my entire understanding of what surgical success could look like.

The truth about ablation versus excision

Let's start with the facts that too many surgeons won't tell you. A 2024 consensus from the World Endometriosis Society finally stated what specialists have known for years: excision surgery is the gold standard for treating endometriosis, especially deep infiltrating disease.

Think of endometriosis lesions like icebergs. What you see on the surface is maybe 10% of what's there. Ablation—burning, vaporizing, or coagulating—only treats that visible tip. Excision cuts out the entire iceberg, including what's hidden beneath.

The numbers tell the story:

- **Ablation**: 80% recurrence rate within 2 years
- **Excision**: 20% recurrence rate at 5 years
- **Multiple ablations**: Each increases scar tissue, making future surgeries harder
- **Proper excision**: Often needs to be done only once

"I had six ablation surgeries between ages 16 and 28," shares Amanda, now 32. "Each one left me worse than before—more scar tissue, more pain. My excision surgery at 29 took seven hours because the surgeon had to work through all that previous damage. But I've been pain-free for three years now. Three years! After a decade of constant agony."

Why most surgeons still do ablation

Here's the uncomfortable truth: excision is harder. Much harder. It requires specialized training that most gynecologists don't have. Ablation takes minutes; excision can take hours. Ablation requires basic laparoscopic skills; excision demands the precision of a microsurgeon.

Dr. Sarah Mitchell, who trained in both techniques, explains: "Imagine trying to peel a sticker off glass. Ablation is like taking a blowtorch to it—quick but messy, leaving residue. Excision is carefully peeling it off intact. Now imagine that sticker is on your intestine, millimeters from vital structures."

The training gap is staggering. Of approximately 52,000 ob-gyns in the US, fewer than 200 are skilled excision specialists. That's less than 0.4%. No wonder women travel across countries— sometimes continents—for proper surgery.

The robotic revolution changing everything

The Hugo™ RAS System hit operating rooms in 2024, and honestly? It's like going from standard definition to 4K Ultra HD. This robotic platform provides 3D visualization with 10x magnification and instruments with seven degrees of freedom— more than the human wrist.

But here's what really matters: the AI integration. The system can detect endometriosis lesions with 97.57% accuracy, highlighting tissue that human eyes might miss. It's like having a second pair of expert eyes that never get tired.

Dr. Kim Lee, who's performed over 100 surgeries with Hugo™, shares the patient impact: "My average surgery time dropped from 4 hours to 2.5 hours. Less time under anesthesia, smaller incisions, faster recovery. But the real win? I'm finding and removing disease I would have missed before. The 3D visualization shows depth and infiltration in ways traditional laparoscopy can't."

The downside? Cost. Robotic surgery adds $3,000-5,000 to surgical fees. Insurance coverage varies wildly. But here's the calculation many women are making: pay more once for surgery likely to work, or pay repeatedly for surgeries that won't?

Preparing your body and mind for surgery

Surgery isn't just what happens in the OR. Success starts weeks before and continues months after. Let me walk you through what actually makes a difference.

Six weeks before surgery

Start here. Not because you need six weeks physically, but because mental preparation takes time.

Anti-inflammatory diet: Reduce surgical inflammation by cutting processed foods, sugar, and alcohol. Increase omega-3s, vegetables, and lean proteins. Maria followed this protocol: "I thought it was woo-woo nonsense. Then my surgeon said my tissue was the 'cleanest' he'd worked with in months. Less inflammation meant easier surgery."

Exercise: Not intense—gentle movement to improve circulation. Walking, swimming, yoga. The goal is blood flow, not fitness gains.

Mental health: Surgery is scary. Period. Find a therapist familiar with medical trauma. Join online support groups. The Endometriosis Association forums have entire sections for pre-surgery anxiety.

Fertility preservation decisions

This conversation should happen before you're on the operating table. If you want biological children someday, consider:

Egg freezing: Optimal before surgery, especially if ovaries are involved. Success rates are age-dependent but improving yearly. Current data shows 46.4% live birth rate from frozen eggs.

Ovarian tissue freezing: For younger women or those who can't delay surgery for egg retrieval. One small piece of ovarian tissue can contain thousands of eggs. When reimplanted later, 90% restore hormone function and 30% achieve pregnancy.

Jessica, 26, shares her decision: "My endometriosis was so aggressive we couldn't delay surgery for egg retrieval. We froze ovarian tissue instead. Knowing it's there, waiting, lets me focus on healing now without fertility panic."

Finding the right surgeon (not just any surgeon)

This might be the most important section you read. The difference between a skilled excision specialist and a general gynecologist doing endometriosis surgery is like the difference between a cardiac surgeon and a general practitioner doing heart surgery. Both might be lovely people. Only one should be operating on you.

Questions that reveal expertise:

1. "How many excision surgeries do you perform annually?" (Look for 50+ minimum)
2. "What's your reoperation rate within 5 years?" (Should be under 20%)
3. "Do you work with a multidisciplinary team?" (Bowel surgeon, urologist on standby)
4. "Can you show me videos of your surgical technique?" (Real specialists are proud to share)
5. "How do you handle endometriosis on the bowel/bladder/diaphragm?" (Should have clear protocols)

Red flags that mean run:

- "Let's try ablation first and see how it goes"
- "You'll need repeat surgeries every few years"
- "I don't operate on the bowel—I'll just remove what I can"
- "Pregnancy will cure your endometriosis"
- "You're too young for such aggressive surgery"
- Unwillingness to discuss technique in detail

The medical tourism option

Let's address this honestly: many women travel for surgery. Not because they want to, but because they have to. Centers of excellence exist globally, often at fraction of US costs.

Romania: Dr. Gabriel Mitroi in Bucharest. Total cost including hospital: €3,000-5,000. Trained at Oxford, specializes in severe cases.

India: Dr. Rooma Sinha in Hyderabad. Pioneered several minimally invasive techniques. Cost: $2,000-4,000 including 5-day hospital stay.

Brazil: Multiple centers in São Paulo. Portuguese-speaking advantage for some. Cost: $3,000-6,000.

But consider hidden costs: travel, accommodation, follow-up care, complications far from home. Sarah traveled to Romania: "Surgery was flawless, saved me $20,000. But when I developed a post-op infection at home, coordinating care between countries was a nightmare."

The surgery itself—what actually happens

Let's demystify the OR. Knowledge reduces fear.

You'll arrive early morning, having fasted since midnight. Pre-op is a blur of consent forms, IV insertion, and marking surgical sites. The anesthesiologist will discuss options—general anesthesia is standard, but some add nerve blocks for better post-op pain control.

In the OR, you're positioned carefully—slight head-down tilt to move intestines away from pelvis. The surgeon makes 3-4 small incisions (5-12mm). Carbon dioxide inflates your abdomen, creating working space. The camera goes in first.

This is where excision diverges from ablation. Instead of burning visible spots, the surgeon systematically examines every surface: reproductive organs, bladder, bowel, peritoneum, even diaphragm in thorough cases. Each lesion is carefully cut out, preserving healthy tissue.

"I watched my surgery video later," shares Keisha. "Four hours condensed to 20 minutes. The precision was incredible—my surgeon removed disease from my ureter while preserving the organ completely. Millimeter by millimeter work."

Recovery reality (not Instagram recovery)

Social media shows women bouncing back in days. Reality? Recovery is a marathon, not a sprint.

Days 1-3: The worst. Gas pain from CO_2 is often worse than incision pain. Walk early and often—shuffling counts. Pain medication is your friend; don't be a hero.

Week 1: Fatigue hits hard. Your body is healing internally even if incisions look good. No lifting, driving, or exercise. Lots of sleeping.

Weeks 2-4: The deceptive phase. You feel better but aren't healed. This is when most complications occur from doing too much. Common mistake: returning to normal activities because you feel "fine."

Months 2-3: True healing phase. Energy returns gradually. Light exercise can resume. Sex might be possible but often uncomfortable initially.

Months 4-6: Assessment phase. This is when you know if surgery was successful. Pain should be significantly reduced or gone.

Lisa documented her recovery: "Day 3: Why did I do this? Week 2: Okay, maybe this will work. Month 3: Oh my god, is this how normal people feel? Month 6: I have my life back."

Complications—the conversation nobody wants but everyone needs

Let's be real about risks. Excision in skilled hands is very safe, but it's still surgery.

Common complications (1-5% rate):

- Infection at incision sites
- Urinary retention requiring temporary catheter
- Constipation from pain meds and slowed digestion
- Emotional crashes from hormone fluctuations

Rare but serious (less than 1% with skilled surgeons):

- Bowel or bladder perforation
- Excessive bleeding requiring transfusion
- Blood clots (prevented by compression devices and early walking)
- Conversion to open surgery

"My bladder was nicked during surgery," shares Rachel. "Sounds terrifying, right? But my surgeon recognized it immediately, repaired it, and kept me catheterized for a week to heal. No long-term damage. This is why you need someone experienced who can handle complications."

Long-term success strategies

Surgery isn't a cure—it's a reset button. Long-term success requires ongoing management.

Hormonal suppression: Many surgeons recommend post-op hormonal therapy to quiet any microscopic disease. This is controversial—some studies show benefit, others don't. Have this discussion based on your individual case.

Pelvic floor therapy: Start 6-8 weeks post-op. Years of pain create muscle dysfunction that surgery alone won't fix. "My surgery removed the disease, but PT taught my muscles how to relax again," explains Maya.

Anti-inflammatory lifestyle: The diet and exercise habits from pre-surgery? Make them permanent. Inflammation feeds endometriosis.

Regular monitoring: Annual ultrasounds or MRIs can catch recurrence early. Some surgeons offer "second look" laparoscopy at 6-12 months for high-risk patients.

The decision tree that guides your choice

Still overwhelmed? Here's your framework:

Choose excision surgery if:

- You have confirmed or suspected endometriosis
- Previous ablations failed
- You have deep infiltrating disease
- Fertility preservation is important
- You can access a skilled specialist

Consider postponing if:

- You're not mentally prepared
- You haven't explored less invasive options
- You can't take adequate recovery time
- You haven't addressed fertility preservation

Seek multiple opinions if:

- Surgeon only offers ablation
- You're told you need a hysterectomy as first-line treatment
- Surgeon won't discuss technique in detail
- You feel rushed or dismissed

Your surgical success toolkit

Pre-op checklist:

- Medical clearance complete
- Time off work arranged (minimum 2 weeks, ideally 4)
- Home prepared (meals prepped, cleaning done)
- Support system activated
- Fertility preservation decided
- Questions for surgeon written down
- Comfortable recovery clothes ready
- Entertainment for recovery downloaded

Recovery milestone tracker:

- Day 1: Out of bed, short walk
- Day 3: Shower independently
- Week 1: Walk around house freely
- Week 2: Short trips outside home
- Week 4: Light activities resume
- Week 6: Exercise clearance
- Week 12: Full activity clearance

Questions for post-op appointment:

- What exactly was found and removed?
- Are pathology results consistent with endometriosis?
- Were all areas of disease addressed?
- What's my recurrence risk?
- Do you recommend suppressive therapy?
- When can I resume normal activities?
- What symptoms warrant immediate contact?

Moving forward with clarity and confidence

As we close this surgical chapter, I want to address the elephant in the room: surgery is scary. It's expensive. Recovery is hard. And there are no guarantees.

But here's what I know after hearing hundreds of surgical stories: the regret comes not from having expert excision surgery, but from waiting too long or settling for inadequate treatment. The women who travel across countries, fight insurance companies, and save for years to access proper surgery? They're not dramatic or excessive. They're informed.

Your surgical journey might be straightforward—find a local specialist, insurance covers it, smooth recovery. Or it might require creativity, persistence, and possibly medical tourism. Either path is valid if it leads to the treatment you deserve.

The woman I was, signing that third surgical consent form through tears? She needed this chapter. She needed to know that her previous surgeries weren't failures of her body but failures of technique. She needed permission to demand better.

You have that permission too.

Coming up in Chapter 6, we're tackling the topic that keeps many women awake at night: fertility. Can you get pregnant with endometriosis? Should you freeze your eggs? What's the real deal with IVF success rates? We'll separate fear from fact and give you a roadmap for whatever family-building journey you choose—including the choice to remain child-free.

Because endometriosis has taken enough from you. It doesn't get to dictate your family planning too.

Chapter 6: Endometriosis and Fertility

The pregnancy test showed two pink lines. After three years of trying, two failed IVF cycles, and one doctor who told me I'd "never conceive naturally with endometriosis this severe," I was staring at proof that sometimes doctors are wrong.

But I'm getting ahead of myself. Let me back up to the day that same doctor delivered my diagnosis, pointing at ultrasound images that looked like a Jackson Pollock painting of adhesions and cysts. "Your chances of natural conception are essentially zero," he said. "Start IVF immediately or consider other options."

I left that appointment devastated. Not just by the endometriosis diagnosis, but by how definitively he'd closed the door on my dreams of motherhood. What I learned over the next three years—through research, second opinions, and connecting with hundreds of women in similar situations—is that fertility with endometriosis is far more nuanced than that black-and-white pronouncement.

The real numbers behind endometriosis and fertility

Let's start with actual data, not doom and gloom. Yes, endometriosis can affect fertility. No, it doesn't mean you're infertile. There's a massive difference between reduced fertility and no fertility, and too many doctors blur that line.

Current research shows:

- **50% of women with mild endometriosis conceive naturally**

- **25% with moderate endometriosis achieve pregnancy without intervention**
- Even with severe endometriosis, **10-15% conceive naturally**

Dr. Maria Santos, who runs one of Europe's largest endometriosis fertility clinics, puts it this way: "I've seen women with minimal endometriosis struggle for years, and women with stage IV disease conceive accidentally. The stage tells us anatomy, not fertility potential."

Age matters more than most doctors emphasize. Under 35 with endometriosis? Your IVF success rates are 95.4%—barely different from women without endo. Over 35? Still 79.6% success rate. Compare that to the general population's age-related decline, and endometriosis adds a hurdle, not a wall.

Here's what changed my perspective entirely: when researchers looked at embryo quality from women with endometriosis, they found something surprising. Once you get good quality embryos, pregnancy rates are 80%—identical to women without endometriosis. The challenge isn't that endometriosis makes you unable to carry a pregnancy. It's that inflammation and anatomy changes can make it harder for egg and sperm to meet, or for an embryo to implant.

Think of it like this: endometriosis doesn't break the baby-making factory. It puts obstacles on the road to the factory.

When preservation becomes your best insurance policy

"I wish someone had talked to me about egg freezing at 28 instead of 38." I've heard versions of this sentence hundreds of times. The cruel irony? Many women don't get diagnosed with endometriosis until their thirties, when egg quantity and quality are already declining.

Current egg freezing technology has revolutionized fertility preservation. The latest data shows a 46.4% live birth rate from frozen eggs—but timing is everything. Here's the breakdown:

- **Under 35**: 10-12 eggs frozen = 70% chance of one live birth
- **35-37**: 15-20 eggs needed for same odds
- **38-40**: 25-30 eggs (often requiring multiple cycles)
- **Over 40**: Success drops significantly

Sarah, diagnosed at 29, made the calculation many women face: "Surgery was urgent—my endometrioma was 8cm and growing. But I wanted kids someday. So we did emergency egg freezing first, surgery six weeks later. Best decision I ever made. Used those eggs at 34 and have twin boys now."

But egg freezing isn't the only option. Ovarian tissue preservation has quietly become a game-changer, especially for younger women. One small strip of ovarian tissue contains thousands of immature eggs. When reimplanted later, 90% of women restore hormone function, and about 30% achieve pregnancy.

The cost variation globally is staggering:

- **Iran**: $1,200 for complete egg freezing cycle
- **Czech Republic**: $2,500 including medications
- **Spain**: $4,000-6,000 with excellent success rates
- **USA**: $15,000-50,000 depending on location and clinic

"I flew to Prague for egg freezing," shares Amanda. "Even with flights and hotels, I spent $4,000 total versus $25,000 quoted in San Francisco. The clinic was actually nicer than the US ones I'd visited."

Making IVF work with endometriosis

If you're heading down the IVF path, know this: standard protocols often need tweaking for endometriosis patients. The inflammation that defines this disease affects every step of the process.

Protocol modifications that improve success:

Low-estrogen approaches: Traditional IVF pumps up estrogen levels, which can flare endometriosis. Many specialists now use letrozole or low-dose stimulation protocols. Lower egg numbers, but better quality and less disease activation.

Frozen transfers only: Fresh transfers happen when your body is inflamed from stimulation. Freezing all embryos and transferring later in a natural or minimally medicated cycle improves success rates by 20-30% in endometriosis patients.

Pre-treatment suppression: Three months of GnRH agonists before IVF seems counterintuitive—why suppress when you're trying to conceive? But studies show it improves egg quality and pregnancy rates, probably by calming inflammation.

Lisa went through four failed standard IVF cycles before switching clinics: "My new doctor said, 'We've been treating you like everyone else. Let's treat your endometriosis first, then help you get pregnant.' Three months of Lupron, then mini-IVF with freeze-all. First frozen transfer worked."

Mini-IVF deserves its own mention. Using minimal stimulation (5-7 eggs instead of 15-20) seems to work better for many endometriosis patients. Less medication, less inflammation, often better outcomes. Dr. John Zhang, who pioneered this approach, reports: "With endometriosis, less is often more. We see better egg quality with gentle stimulation."

The emotional minefield nobody prepares you for

Can we talk about the mental load? Fertility challenges with endometriosis create a special kind of hell. You're grieving your health AND your fertility. You're managing chronic pain while injecting yourself with hormones. You're broke from treatments and exhausted from fighting.

"I became someone I didn't recognize," admits Jennifer. "Obsessed with ovulation tests, devastated by every period, angry at every pregnancy announcement. My therapist said I was grieving—not just the pregnancies that didn't happen, but the easy conception I'd always imagined."

The stats back this up: women undergoing fertility treatment with endometriosis have 2.5 times higher rates of depression and anxiety than those with other infertility causes.

What helps:

- **Specialized therapy**: Find someone who understands both chronic illness and infertility
- **Medication if needed**: Antidepressants won't affect your fertility
- **Support groups**: But choose carefully—some can become toxic positivity or competition zones
- **Treatment breaks**: Sometimes stepping back saves your sanity and your relationship

When plans A, B, and C don't work

Let's be real—not every fertility story has a baby at the end. And that's okay. Actually, it's more than okay. The pressure to keep trying can become its own trauma.

Surrogacy offers a path when carrying a pregnancy isn't possible or advisable. Global options vary wildly:

- **Ukraine**: $30,000-40,000 total cost, clear legal framework
- **Greece**: $40,000-50,000, EU standards of care
- **USA**: $100,000-150,000, strongest legal protections
- **Canada**: Altruistic only (no payment beyond expenses)

Rachel chose surrogacy after five years of failed treatments: "My body was done. I was done. Using a surrogate let me become a mother without destroying what was left of my health."

Adoption remains a beautiful way to build a family, though endometriosis can complicate the process. Some agencies require medical clearance that your condition won't affect parenting ability. International adoption may have fewer health restrictions than domestic infant adoption.

Single parenthood by choice is increasingly common. Emma, 37, decided to pursue motherhood solo: "Waiting for a partner while my fertility declined felt like letting endometriosis control another part of my life. I used donor sperm, did IVF, and have zero regrets."

Choosing child-free life deserves equal respect and validation. The constant "when are you having kids?" questions hit differently when the answer involves medical trauma.

"I spent six years and $80,000 trying to have a baby," shares Christina. "One day I realized I was trying to prove endometriosis couldn't win. But choosing to stop wasn't letting it win—it was choosing my life back. I'm genuinely happy child-free now."

Your fertility decision framework

Facing fertility decisions with endometriosis feels overwhelming. Here's a framework that's helped hundreds of women find clarity:

Step 1: Medical inventory

- Current disease status (recent imaging)
- Ovarian reserve testing (AMH, FSH, antral follicle count)
- Partner's fertility status (don't assume it's all you)
- Overall health beyond endometriosis

Step 2: Life inventory

- Financial resources (including potential for loans/grants)
- Relationship stability
- Career flexibility
- Support system strength
- Mental health baseline

Step 3: Values clarification

- Is genetic connection important?
- How do you feel about medical intervention?
- What does family mean to you?
- How much are you willing to sacrifice?

Step 4: Timeline creation

- Immediate options (next 6 months)
- Short-term plan (1-2 years)
- Long-term possibilities (2-5 years)
- Stop points (when to reassess)

Financial resources that actually help

Money shouldn't determine who gets to be a parent, but it does. Here are resources that can help:

Grants:

- **Baby Quest**: Up to $15,000 for IVF
- **Tinina Q. Cade Foundation**: $10,000 grants
- **Family Reach**: Financial assistance during treatment
- **International grants**: Many countries have specific programs

Creative funding:

- Fertility loans (careful—interest rates vary)
- Employer benefits (more companies covering fertility)
- Clinical trials (free treatment in exchange for participation)
- Crowdfunding (average raises $3,000-5,000)
- Treatment abroad (even with travel, often cheaper)

Your fertility preservation calculator

Let's get practical. Here's how to calculate your real costs:

Egg freezing:

- Base cost: $6,000-15,000
- Medications: $3,000-5,000
- Storage: $500-1,000/year
- Future use (thaw, fertilize, transfer): $5,000-8,000
- Total investment: $15,000-30,000

IVF with endometriosis:

- Expect 1.5x cycles compared to other diagnoses
- Additional medications for suppression
- Possible surgical prep

- Frozen transfers add $3,000-5,000 each
- Realistic total: $30,000-60,000

Alternative paths:

- Surrogacy: $30,000-150,000
- Adoption: $20,000-45,000
- Donor eggs: $25,000-35,000
- Living child-free: $0 (but therapy recommended)

The hope I want to leave you with

That positive pregnancy test I mentioned at the start? It came after I'd given up. Not given up on being a mother, but given up on forcing my body to perform on my timeline. I'd had excision surgery, done acupuncture, changed my diet, tried three IUIs. Then I took a break. Six months of no temperature charting, no ovulation tests, no timed intercourse.

That's when it happened.

I'm not saying "just relax and it'll happen"—that's toxic positivity garbage. What I'm saying is that fertility with endometriosis rarely follows the path we plan. Your journey might include IVF, or adoption, or surrogacy, or choosing child-free life. All are valid. All can lead to happiness.

What matters is that you make decisions from a place of information, not fear. That you understand your real options, not just worst-case scenarios. That you give yourself permission to change course if needed.

Endometriosis complicates fertility. That's fact. But complicated doesn't mean impossible. And even when biological motherhood isn't possible, meaningful, joyful life is always within reach.

Coming up in Chapter 7, we'll explore lifestyle strategies that actually help—not the "just do yoga" nonsense, but evidence-based approaches to managing symptoms and improving quality of life. Because whatever your fertility journey looks like, you deserve to feel as good as possible along the way.

Chapter 7: Lifestyle and Self-Help Strategies

My acupuncturist stuck the thirteenth needle into my abdomen, and I finally broke. Not from pain—the needles barely register compared to endometriosis. I broke from exhaustion. Three years of trying everything: elimination diets, supplements, yoga, meditation, essential oils, energy healing, and now this. My credit cards were maxed, my hope was shot, and I still hurt every single day.

"How many more sessions?" I asked through tears.

She paused, then said something that changed my entire approach: "You're collecting treatments like Pokemon cards, hoping one will be the magic cure. What if instead, we built you a sustainable system using only what actually works?"

That conversation led me down a research rabbit hole that transformed how I manage endometriosis. Turns out, there's solid science behind some complementary therapies—and absolutely none behind others. The trick is knowing the difference.

The complementary therapies that actually work

Let's cut through the wellness industry BS and talk evidence. Because while your aunt's friend swears that crystal healing cured her endo, you deserve treatments backed by actual research.

Acupuncture leads the pack. Multiple systematic reviews show consistent results: average pain reduction of 1.36 points on a 10-point scale. That might not sound like much, but when you're living at an 8, dropping to a 6.5 makes the difference between bedridden and functional.

The mechanism makes sense too. Acupuncture reduces inflammatory markers, modulates pain perception, and may influence hormone regulation. An 81% pain reduction rate in one major study isn't placebo effect—it's legitimate therapeutic intervention.

Maria's experience mirrors the research: "I was skeptical as hell. Lying there with needles in me, thinking about the $80 I was wasting. But after six weeks, twice-weekly sessions, I had my first pain-free period in five years. Not low pain. NO pain."

But here's the catch—practitioner quality matters enormously. Look for:

- Licensed acupuncturist (L.Ac.) credentials
- Specific training in gynecological conditions
- Experience with endometriosis patients
- Clean, professional clinic setting

Pelvic floor physical therapy might be the most underutilized treatment for endometriosis. Years of pain create muscle dysfunction—your pelvic floor literally forgets how to relax. Expert consensus strongly supports PT as essential complementary treatment.

"I thought PT was for incontinence after babies," admits Jessica. "But my therapist explained that my muscles were in constant spasm from guarding against pain. Eight weeks of internal work, breathing exercises, and home stretches reduced my daily pain by 60%."

What happens in pelvic floor PT:

- Internal and external muscle assessment

- Trigger point release
- Breathing coordination
- Postural correction
- Home exercise program
- Sometimes biofeedback or electrical stimulation

TENS units (transcutaneous electrical nerve stimulation) showed positive results in randomized controlled trials. Participants using TENS for 20 minutes twice daily reported significant pain reduction compared to placebo. At $30-100 for a unit you own forever, it's accessible pain relief.

Mindfulness-based stress reduction (MBSR) proved especially effective when delivered virtually. An 8-week online program reduced pain scores, improved quality of life, and decreased anxiety in endometriosis patients. The virtual format meant participants could practice from bed during flares—practical adaptation at its finest.

What the science says about your plate

Every wellness influencer has an endometriosis diet to sell you. Most are nonsense. But legitimate research does support specific nutritional approaches.

The **Mediterranean diet** consistently shows benefits. Not because it's magical, but because it's naturally anti-inflammatory. High in omega-3s, antioxidants, and fiber while low in processed foods and red meat—everything that research suggests helps manage inflammatory conditions.

Let me break down what actually has evidence:

Omega-3 fatty acids: Women consuming the highest amounts had 22% lower risk of endometriosis. For those already diagnosed, 1-2 grams daily of fish oil reduced inflammatory markers and pain scores. Food sources work too—fatty fish twice weekly, walnuts, chia seeds, ground flax.

N-acetylcysteine (NAC): Remember from Chapter 4? This supplement deserves repeating. 600mg three times daily shrank endometriomas in multiple studies. It's one of the few supplements with strong enough evidence that surgeons recommend it (Italian Multicenter Trial, 2023).

Curcumin: The active compound in turmeric reduced endometriotic lesions in animal studies and improved pain in human trials. But—and this is crucial—you need it with black pepper (piperine) for absorption. 500-1000mg twice daily with meals.

The elimination diet debate

Here's where things get controversial. A 2023 Italian study found 52% of endometriosis patients improved on a gluten-free diet (Marziali et al., 2023). But before you throw out all your bread, understand the nuance.

The improvement likely comes from:

- Reduced overall inflammation (gluten can be inflammatory for some)
- Eating less processed food (most gluten-free diets force whole food choices)
- Placebo effect (feeling in control helps)
- Possible undiagnosed celiac disease (more common in endo patients)

Sarah tried everything: "Gluten-free for six months—no change. Dairy-free—maybe slightly better? But when I cut ultra-processed foods and added more vegetables, that's when my energy improved and bloating decreased."

My advice? Try elimination diets systematically:

1. Keep a detailed food and symptom diary for 2 weeks baseline
2. Eliminate one category for 4-6 weeks
3. Reintroduce slowly, noting any changes
4. Only continue restrictions that show clear benefit

Common eliminations to try:

- Gluten
- Dairy
- Red meat
- Alcohol
- High FODMAP foods (if you have GI symptoms)
- Added sugars

Movement that helps, not hurts

"Just exercise!" ranks right up there with "just relax!" in useless endometriosis advice. But specific types of movement, done correctly, can genuinely help.

A 2025 systematic review finally gave us clear data: exercise improves quality of life in endometriosis patients, but the type and intensity matter enormously.

Yoga emerged as the winner, specifically Hatha yoga practiced for 90 minutes twice weekly. Studies show reduced pain, improved flexibility, and better mental health outcomes. The key? Modifications during flares and avoiding inversions during menstruation.

Lisa found her sweet spot: "Power yoga made everything worse—too much core work aggravated my adhesions. But gentle Hatha with lots of hip openers and restorative poses? Game changer. I can tell when I skip a week."

Swimming offers unique benefits. The buoyancy reduces joint stress while water pressure provides gentle abdominal support. Many women report swimming as the only exercise tolerable during flares. Warm water pools (84-88°F) work best—cold can trigger cramping.

Strength training requires careful modification:

- Avoid heavy core work during flares
- Focus on posterior chain (back, glutes, hamstrings)
- Use lighter weights with more repetitions
- Stop any exercise that triggers pain
- Work with trainers familiar with chronic pain

"I mourned giving up CrossFit," shares Amanda. "But working with a trainer who understood endometriosis, I built a program that actually reduced my pain. Strengthening my back and glutes took pressure off my pelvis."

Ancient wisdom meets modern science

The integration of traditional medicine systems with conventional treatment shows promising results, but requires careful navigation.

Traditional Chinese Medicine (TCM) views endometriosis as "blood stagnation" with underlying patterns of cold, heat, or deficiency. While the terminology sounds unscientific, the treatments often align with current understanding of inflammation and circulation.

Beyond acupuncture, TCM practitioners might recommend:

- Herbal formulas (some show legitimate anti-inflammatory effects)
- Dietary therapy based on food "temperatures"
- Qi gong or tai chi for gentle movement

- Moxibustion for specific symptoms

Ayurveda approaches endometriosis through the lens of doshas and tissue health. Panchakarma—a detoxification protocol—showed benefits in small studies, though larger trials are needed. What's interesting is how Ayurvedic dietary recommendations often mirror anti-inflammatory protocols.

Priya integrated both systems: "My Ayurvedic practitioner had me eat warming foods and avoid cold drinks—which sounded weird until I noticed less bloating. Combined with conventional treatment, these small changes added up."

Indigenous practices vary globally but often emphasize plant medicines and ceremony. While research is limited, the psychological benefits of cultural connection and ritual shouldn't be dismissed. Just ensure any herbs don't interact with medications.

Safety first—the integration checklist

Combining conventional and complementary treatments requires coordination. Use this checklist:

Before starting any new therapy:

- Tell all providers about all treatments
- Check herb-drug interactions
- Start one new thing at a time
- Track results objectively
- Set realistic expectations
- Have a stop point if it's not working

Red flags to avoid:

- Anyone promising a "cure"
- Pressure to stop conventional treatment

- Extremely expensive protocols
- Lack of professional credentials
- Unwillingness to work with your doctor

Your personalized lifestyle toolkit

One-size-fits-all doesn't work with endometriosis. Build your toolkit based on your symptoms, budget, and life.

Weekly Lifestyle Planner Template:

Monday: Acupuncture (if in treatment cycle), meal prep anti-inflammatory dinners *Tuesday*: Gentle yoga, supplement check-in *Wednesday*: Pelvic PT or self-massage, batch cook lunches *Thursday*: Rest day if needed, or light swimming *Friday*: Acupuncture, grocery shop for next week *Weekend*: Longer yoga session, social activities planned around energy

Supplement Safety Checker:

- NAC: Check kidney function first, avoid with nitroglycerin
- Omega-3s: Can thin blood, careful with other anticoagulants
- Curcumin: May interact with diabetes medications
- Probiotics: Generally safe but quality varies wildly
- Vitamin D: Test levels first, toxicity possible with high doses

Exercise Modifications by Symptoms:

High pain days: Gentle stretching, breathing exercises, short walks *Moderate pain*: Swimming, restorative yoga, light resistance bands *Low pain*: Full yoga practice, moderate strength training, longer walks *Pain-free*: Whatever brings you joy—dance, hike, bike

Finding qualified practitioners:

Questions to ask:

1. "How many endometriosis patients have you treated?"
2. "What's your success rate with pelvic pain?"
3. "How do you coordinate with medical doctors?"
4. "What's your training background?"
5. "How many sessions typically needed?"

Green flags:

- Specific experience with endometriosis
- Realistic expectations
- Willing to communicate with your medical team
- Clear pricing structure
- Professional boundaries

The honest truth about lifestyle changes

After all this information, here's what I need you to understand: lifestyle modifications aren't a cure. They're tools. Really good tools that can significantly improve your quality of life, but tools nonetheless.

You might do everything "right"—perfect anti-inflammatory diet, regular acupuncture, daily yoga—and still have bad days. That's not failure. That's endometriosis.

What lifestyle changes offer is agency. Instead of feeling helpless against pain, you have options. Instead of waiting for the next medical appointment, you have daily practices that help. Instead of your body feeling like the enemy, you develop partnership.

"I spent years angry that lifestyle changes didn't cure me," reflects Carmen. "Then I realized—my daily yoga practice meant I used 50% less pain medication. My diet changes reduced bloating from unbearable to manageable. Acupuncture gave me two good weeks each month instead of one. That's not failure. That's reclaiming half my life."

Your next steps

As we move toward Chapter 8 on coping with chronic pain, take inventory. What from this chapter resonates? What seems worth trying? What definitely doesn't fit your life?

Start small. Pick one evidence-based therapy and commit to a fair trial—at least 6-8 weeks. Track results objectively. If it helps, keep it. If not, try something else. This isn't about perfection; it's about building a life that works with endometriosis, not against it.

The woman crying on the acupuncture table three years ago? She found her system. Acupuncture twice monthly for maintenance. Swimming three times a week. Mediterranean-style eating most days. NAC and omega-3s daily. Yoga when energy allows. Is she cured? No. Is she living fully? Absolutely.

Your system will look different. But with evidence as your guide and patience as your companion, you'll find what works. Chapter 8 will help you handle the days when even the best system isn't enough—because those days come too, and that's okay.

Chapter 8: Coping with Chronic Pain

The pain hit at 3 AM, ripping me from sleep like a fire alarm in my pelvis. I knew this dance. Stumble to the bathroom. Vomit from pain intensity. Curl on the cold floor because somehow the tiles help. Wait for pain meds to maybe work. Count the minutes until dawn.

But this night was different. This night, I finally understood something my pain psychologist had been trying to tell me for months: "Your nervous system is like a security alarm. With endometriosis, the alarm becomes oversensitive—even small problems trigger a loud alarm. Sometimes it keeps going even after the problem is fixed."

Lying there on those bathroom tiles, I realized my body had been screaming "DANGER!" for so long that it forgot how to turn off the alarm. Even when the endometriosis was treated, my nervous system kept sounding the siren. That revelation changed everything about how I approached pain management.

Your pain is real, and your brain is trying to help

Let's get something straight right now. The pain-brain connection doesn't mean your pain is "all in your head." It means your brain and nervous system are doing exactly what they're designed to do—protect you from perceived threats. The problem is, with chronic pain, the system gets stuck in overdrive.

Think of it this way: if you touch a hot stove, pain signals race to your brain, you jerk your hand back, crisis averted. But with endometriosis, it's like your nervous system thinks you're touching that hot stove 24/7. Your brain, trying to be helpful, amplifies every signal, creates new pain pathways, and basically turns into an overprotective helicopter parent.

Dr. Sarah Chen's research on chronic pain explains it perfectly: "Chronic pain actually changes brain structure. Areas responsible for pain processing become hyperactive while areas managing pain suppression shrink. It's not psychological—it's neurological remodeling".

This is why you might still hurt after successful surgery. Why stress makes pain worse. Why that random Tuesday might be agony while the day you expected pain isn't so bad. Your nervous system is running its own show, and it needs different management than acute pain.

Evidence-based strategies that actually work

After years of "have you tried yoga?" and "just think positive!" advice, let's talk about what research actually supports for chronic pain management.

Cognitive Behavioral Therapy (CBT) for chronic pain tops the evidence list. A 2024 systematic review found CBT reduced pain intensity, improved function, and decreased depression in chronic pain patients. But we're not talking about generic therapy—this is specialized CBT that targets pain catastrophizing, fear avoidance, and activity pacing.

"I thought therapy for pain was ridiculous," admits Rachel. "I have actual tissue damage! But my pain psychologist taught me to recognize when I was catastrophizing—turning 'this hurts' into 'this will never end and my life is over.' Learning to catch and challenge those thoughts literally reduced my pain levels."

What happens in pain-focused CBT:

- Identify pain triggers and patterns
- Challenge catastrophic thinking
- Develop coping statements that work
- Learn activity pacing (huge for endometriosis)
- Build behavioral strategies for flares

Heat therapy seems basic, but specific protocols maximize benefit. Research shows 15-20 minutes of heat at 104-113°F (40-45°C) reduces muscle tension and increases blood flow. But timing matters—apply at the first sign of cramping, not after pain peaks.

Lisa discovered this accidentally: "I was using heat for hours, wondering why it stopped helping. My physical therapist explained that after 20 minutes, you're just irritating tissue. Now I do 20 on, 40 off, repeat. Way more effective."

Breathing techniques actually change pain perception. Not woo-woo "breathe through it" nonsense, but specific patterns that activate the parasympathetic nervous system:

Box breathing: Inhale 4 counts, hold 4, exhale 4, hold 4. Repeat 4-8 cycles. Navy SEALs use this for stress—it works for pain too.

4-7-8 method: Inhale 4, hold 7, exhale 8. This activates the vagus nerve, reducing inflammation and pain signals.

"Breathing exercises made me angry at first," shares Maria. "Like I could breathe away endometriosis! But using them preventively—every morning, before stressful events—reduced my baseline pain. It's not about breathing through active pain; it's about calming the system before it spirals."

Progressive muscle relaxation showed significant benefit in multiple studies. The key is regular practice when you're NOT in pain, training your body to release tension on command. Start with guided audio, eventually you'll do it automatically.

The mental health connection nobody prepared you for

Here's a truth bomb: 80-86.5% of endometriosis patients experience depression. 80-87.5% have anxiety. These aren't separate issues—they're part of the same inflammatory process affecting your brain.

Recent research revealed shared genetic factors between endometriosis and psychiatric conditions. The same genes that predispose you to endo also increase risk for depression and anxiety. Add chronic pain, medical trauma, and life disruption? Your mental health challenges aren't weakness—they're biology plus circumstance.

"I spent years thinking I was going crazy," reflects Jennifer. "Panic attacks, depression spirals, feeling disconnected from my body. Learning that endometriosis causes actual brain inflammation validated everything. I wasn't weak. My brain was literally inflamed."

PTSD from medical trauma is real and common. Years of dismissal, painful procedures, failed treatments—these create genuine trauma. EMDR (Eye Movement Desensitization and Reprocessing) therapy shows particular effectiveness for medical trauma, helping process those experiences without re-traumatizing.

Signs of medical PTSD:

- Panic attacks before appointments
- Avoiding necessary medical care
- Flashbacks to painful procedures
- Hypervigilance about body sensations
- Emotional numbing during exams

Crisis resources when it's too much

Sometimes you need help RIGHT NOW. Here are global resources:

USA:

- National Suicide Prevention Lifeline: 988
- Crisis Text Line: Text HOME to 741741
- SAMHSA National Helpline: 1-800-662-4357

UK:

- Samaritans: 116 123
- Mind Infoline: 0300 123 3393
- Text SHOUT to 85258

Canada:

- Talk Suicide Canada: 1-833-456-4566
- Text 45645

Australia:

- Lifeline: 13 11 14
- Beyond Blue: 1300 22 4636

International:

- findahelpline.com (directory for 60+ countries)
- WhatsApp crisis lines available in many countries

Building your personalized pain toolkit

One size doesn't fit all with pain management. You need a toolkit with options for different situations.

The Flare-Up Action Plan

Create this when you're calm, use it when you're not:

Level 1 (early warning signs):

- Preemptive heat therapy
- Gentle stretching routine
- Cancel non-essential plans
- Start anti-inflammatory diet

Level 2 (escalating pain):

- Medication per protocol
- TENS unit application
- Breathing exercises
- Contact support person

Level 3 (severe pain):

- Emergency medication
- All comfort measures
- Decision point: ER or ride it out?
- Activate emergency support

Level 4 (crisis):

- Emergency room protocol
- Pre-written medical history
- Support person takes over
- No decision-making alone

Communication strategies for invisible pain

Explaining pain nobody can see is exhausting. Develop scripts:

For family: "My pain today is a 7. That means I can participate in X but not Y. I need help with Z."

For work: "I'm experiencing a symptom flare of my chronic condition. I can manage priority tasks A and B remotely but need to postpone C."

For doctors: "My baseline pain is typically 4-5. Today is 8. This is different because [specific changes]. I've tried [interventions] without relief."

For doubters: "I understand my pain isn't visible. Endometriosis causes internal inflammation and nerve dysfunction. Would you like resources to understand better?"

Medication management without dependence

Chronic pain often means long-term medication, raising addiction concerns. Evidence-based strategies for safe use:

- Work with pain specialists, not just gynecologists
- Use multimodal approach (never rely on one medication)
- Scheduled dosing vs. as-needed for baseline pain
- Regular medication reviews and tolerance breaks
- Non-opioid options first, always
- Track effectiveness objectively

"I was terrified of becoming addicted," shares Amanda. "But my pain doctor explained the difference between dependence (physical) and addiction (behavioral). With proper monitoring and multiple strategies, I've used the same low dose for three years effectively."

Alternative approaches with actual evidence

Beyond mainstream medicine, some alternatives show promise:

Medical cannabis: Where legal, specific CBD:THC ratios help some patients. Start low, track carefully, work with knowledgeable providers.

Ketamine therapy: Low-dose ketamine infusions show promise for chronic pain, especially with central sensitization. Expensive but life-changing for some.

Neurofeedback: Training your brain waves sounds sci-fi, but studies support effectiveness for chronic pain. Requires multiple sessions but provides lasting benefit.

What doesn't work (save your money):

- Magnetic jewelry
- Most detox protocols
- Alkaline water
- Colon cleanses
- Energy healing (unless placebo effect helps you)

Your practical pain tracking system

Effective pain management requires data. Use this template:

Daily tracking (scale 1-10):

- Morning pain level
- Afternoon pain level
- Evening pain level
- Sleep quality
- Medication effectiveness
- Triggers identified
- Helpful interventions

Weekly patterns:

- Best/worst days

- Menstrual cycle correlation
- Stress level impact
- Activity correlation
- Weather sensitivity

Monthly analysis:

- Overall trajectory
- Medication adjustments needed
- Strategy effectiveness
- Quality of life measures

"Tracking revealed patterns I missed," notes Caroline. "Tuesday staff meetings always triggered Wednesday flares. Turns out, sitting in those awful chairs for two hours was the culprit. Got accommodation for a different chair—Wednesday pain reduced by 40%."

Mental health screening that matters

Regular mental health check-ins are as important as physical monitoring. Use validated tools:

PHQ-9 for depression: Score above 10? Time for professional support.

GAD-7 for anxiety: Score above 10? Anxiety needs addressing.

PC-PTSD-5 for trauma: Any "yes" answers? Consider trauma-informed therapy.

Do these monthly. Catching mental health changes early prevents spirals.

Living fully with chronic pain

Here's what I know after years of wrestling with chronic pain: it's not about winning or losing. It's about learning to dance with a really difficult partner.

Some days, pain leads and you follow. Other days, you take charge. Most days fall somewhere between. The goal isn't pain-free living—though that would be nice. The goal is rich, meaningful life despite pain.

"I grieved my pain-free self for years," reflects Diana. "Then I realized—that person is gone. This person, who manages pain daily, who's learned incredible resilience, who appreciates good days deeply—she's pretty amazing too."

Your path forward

Chapter 9 awaits, where we'll tackle the practical realities of work, school, and relationships with endometriosis. Because managing pain is one thing—managing life while managing pain requires its own strategies.

But for now, acknowledge what you've learned. Your pain is real. Your brain is doing its best. You have more tools than you realized. And tomorrow, you'll add more to your toolkit.

That 3 AM bathroom floor awakening? It still happens sometimes. But now I have heat packs staged strategically, meditation apps downloaded, support people on speed dial, and most importantly—understanding that my overprotective nervous system needs compassion, not combat.

Your journey with chronic pain is uniquely yours. But you're not walking it alone.

Chapter 9: Work, School, and Relationships

The email from HR sat in my inbox like a ticking bomb. "Re: Your Recent Absences." Three months into my dream job, and I was already flagged as a "problem employee." Never mind my excellent performance reviews or the projects I'd completed ahead of schedule. Missing eight days in three months—all for endometriosis flares—apparently trumped everything else.

I had two choices: hide my condition and hope for the best, or disclose and request accommodations. Neither felt safe. But then I met Sarah at an endometriosis support group. She'd successfully navigated workplace accommodations for five years. "The law is on your side," she said, "but you need to know how to use it."

That conversation changed my professional life. And personal life. And financial future. Because here's what nobody tells you: endometriosis doesn't just affect your uterus. It affects every single aspect of how you move through the world.

Your rights are stronger than you think

Most women with endometriosis don't realize they have legal protections. Let's fix that right now.

In the **United States**, the Americans with Disabilities Act (ADA) covers endometriosis when it substantially limits major life activities. That includes working, concentrating, sleeping, and reproductive functions. The 2008 amendments made coverage broader—you don't need to be completely disabled to qualify.

The **UK's Equality Act 2010** protects against discrimination for any physical impairment with substantial, long-term adverse effects on daily activities. Endometriosis qualifies. Full stop. MPs have specifically addressed this in Parliament, noting that employers must make reasonable adjustments.

Canada's Human Rights Act and provincial codes prohibit discrimination based on disability, which includes chronic conditions like endometriosis. Each province has slightly different processes, but federal protections apply everywhere.

Australia's Disability Discrimination Act covers chronic illness that affects daily life. Fair Work Australia has ruled in favor of endometriosis accommodations multiple times.

But knowing your rights and using them? Two different things.

Workplace accommodations that actually help

"Reasonable accommodation" sounds vague because it's meant to be flexible. What works depends on your job, symptoms, and employer. Here's what's actually helped real women:

Flexible scheduling: Start times that accommodate morning symptoms, ability to shift hours during flares, compressed work weeks during good periods.

Jessica negotiated this beautifully: "I proposed working 10-hour days when I feel good, banking time for flare days. My productivity actually increased because I wasn't forcing myself to work through severe pain."

Remote work options: Not full-time necessarily, but the ability to work from home during flares. This became easier post-2020, but some employers are rolling back flexibility.

"I can do my job curled up with a heating pad," explains Monica. "The only difference is I'm not pretending to be fine in the office. My work quality stays consistent."

Ergonomic support: Standing desks, supportive chairs, footrests, proximity to bathrooms, private spaces for emergency rest.

Modified duties: Temporary adjustment of physical requirements, deadline flexibility during known difficult periods (like menstruation), job-sharing arrangements.

Leave accommodations: Intermittent FMLA in the US, sick leave policies that don't penalize chronic conditions, ability to make up time rather than use PTO.

The key? Proposing solutions, not just presenting problems.

How to request accommodations without tanking your career

Here's your strategic approach:

Step 1: Document everything Before disclosure, track your symptoms, work impact, and how accommodations would help. Use specific metrics: "I miss an average of 2 days monthly but could reduce this to 0.5 days with work-from-home options."

Step 2: Know your company's process Large companies have formal ADA coordinators. Small companies might handle it through HR or directly with your manager. Get the process in writing.

Step 3: Prepare your initial disclosure Keep it professional and solution-focused. You don't need to share gruesome details.

Sample script: "I have a chronic medical condition that occasionally affects my ability to work on-site. I'm requesting reasonable accommodations to maintain my high performance level. I've prepared some proposals that wouldn't affect my core job duties."

Step 4: Get medical documentation Your doctor needs to confirm you have a condition requiring accommodation but shouldn't disclose specifics unless necessary. Use this template:

"[Patient] has a chronic gynecological condition that substantially limits major life activities. Recommended accommodations include: [specific list]. These accommodations would enable the patient to perform essential job functions effectively."

Step 5: Negotiate in good faith Your employer can propose alternatives if your requests cause "undue hardship." Be flexible but don't accept discriminatory alternatives.

Success story time: Rachel, a marketing manager, requested work-from-home twice monthly. Her company countered with one day monthly. She negotiated for "as-needed with 24-hour notice when possible, not to exceed 4 days monthly." Both sides won.

When education becomes a battlefield

Educational settings create unique challenges. You're paying to be there, but still need to show up. Here's how to navigate:

For US students, two laws matter:

504 Plans (K-12): Requires accommodations for students with disabilities in public schools. Endometriosis qualifies when it impacts learning.

Common accommodations:

- Bathroom passes without question
- Ability to stand/move during class
- Extended time for assignments during flares
- Excused absences with makeup work
- Access to nurse's office for medication

IEPs (Individualized Education Programs): For students whose condition significantly impacts educational performance. More comprehensive than 504 plans.

"My daughter's 504 plan saved her education," shares Patricia. "Stop-the-clock testing for bathroom breaks, permission to wear heating pads, and flexible PE requirements. She went from failing to honor roll."

University students have different protections through disability services offices. Every university has one—use it.

Standard accommodations:

- Priority registration (schedule around symptoms)
- Flexible attendance policies
- Extended test time
- Ability to take breaks during exams
- Note-taking assistance
- Remote learning options when needed

International approaches vary:

- **UK**: Disabled Students' Allowance provides funding for accommodations
- **Canada**: Provincial funding and university-specific programs
- **Australia**: Disability support services plus government assistance

The trick? Register BEFORE you need help. Mid-crisis is the worst time to navigate bureaucracy.

Relationships in the time of chronic pain

Let's be honest—endometriosis tests every relationship you have. Romantic partners, family, friends, colleagues. Some rise to the challenge. Others... don't.

Partner communication that works

"My pain isn't about you" might be the most important sentence you'll ever say. Partners often feel helpless, rejected, or even blamed when chronic illness affects intimacy and plans.

Emma developed this approach: "I rate my symptoms daily on a shared app. Green days mean I'm up for anything. Yellow means proceed with caution. Red means survival mode. It removes the constant 'how are you feeling?' questions and helps him understand patterns."

Scripts for difficult conversations:

About cancelled plans: "I'm as disappointed as you are. This isn't what I choose. Let's reschedule for [specific date] and have a backup plan."

About intimacy: "I want to be close to you. Right now, penetration causes pain, but [specific alternatives] would feel good. Can we explore what works for both of us?"

About future concerns: "I know my condition creates uncertainty. Let's talk about our fears and plans realistically. What do you need to know to feel secure?"

Dyspareunia solutions nobody talks about

Painful sex affects 64% of women with endometriosis, but it's treatable. Options beyond "just relax":

- Pelvic floor physical therapy (often covered by insurance)
- Vaginal dilators with proper guidance
- Position modifications (you on top = more control)
- Extended foreplay for natural lubrication
- High-quality lubricants (silicone-based last longer)
- Non-penetrative intimacy options
- Treatment of specific trigger points
- Hormone therapy for vaginal tissues

"We mourned 'normal' sex for months," admits Lisa. "Then we discovered that taking penetration off the table temporarily led to the most creative, connected intimacy we'd ever had. When penetration became possible again, our entire sexual relationship had improved."

Family dynamics across cultures

Cultural context massively impacts family support. In collectivist cultures, family involvement can be overwhelming. In individualist cultures, you might struggle alone.

Maria navigates her Mexican family: "They want to help but think prayer and herbs cure everything. I appreciate their love while maintaining boundaries about medical decisions."

Amara deals with different challenges in her Nigerian family: "Endometriosis affects fertility, which is everything in my culture. I had to educate them that pressure to conceive actually worsens my condition."

Strategies that help:

- Designate one family spokesperson to reduce repetitive conversations
- Provide educational materials in appropriate languages
- Set boundaries about medical advice
- Include supportive family members in medical appointments
- Create rituals that honor both culture and medical needs

Teaching friends without lecturing

Your social circle needs education, but nobody wants a medical lecture at brunch.

Quick education wins:

- Share one specific impact: "Endometriosis makes me cancel plans last-minute sometimes. It's not personal."
- Use analogies: "Imagine appendicitis-level pain, but monthly and doctors don't believe you."
- Redirect Google warriors: "I appreciate you caring. I'm working with specialists on treatment."
- Be specific about help: "Checking in without expecting responses really helps" vs. "Be supportive."

Financial survival with chronic illness

Endometriosis is expensive. Between medical costs, lost wages, and career impacts, financial planning becomes crucial.

Insurance maximization strategies:

- Appeal every denial (success rate increases with each appeal)
- Get case managers for complex situations
- Use patient advocates when available
- Track every expense for tax deductions
- Understand your out-of-pocket maximum

- Time procedures strategically within plan years

"I scheduled surgery for January to hit my deductible early," shares Amanda. "Then packed all other procedures into that year. Saved thousands."

Disability benefits navigation

The US Social Security Disability Insurance (SSDI) process is notoriously difficult, but endometriosis can qualify when:

- You can't work any job (not just your current one)
- Condition has lasted/will last 12+ months
- Medical documentation is extensive

Tips from successful applicants:

- File immediately upon work cessation
- Get a disability attorney (they're paid from back benefits)
- Document everything—pain levels, failed treatments, work attempts
- Include mental health impacts
- Appeal denials (most are initially denied)

Other countries' systems:

- **UK**: Personal Independence Payment (PIP) for daily living costs
- **Canada**: Canada Pension Plan disability benefits
- **Australia**: Disability Support Pension through Centrelink

Self-employment as solution and challenge

Many women with endometriosis turn to self-employment for flexibility. But it's not all freedom and yoga pants.

Advantages:

- Complete schedule control
- No accommodation negotiations
- Work from bed when needed
- Build around symptoms

Challenges:

- No paid sick leave
- Expensive individual health insurance
- Inconsistent income during flares
- Self-employment tax burden
- Isolation during illness

"Freelancing saved my sanity but challenged my finances," reflects Stephanie. "I learned to charge higher rates to cover sick days, save aggressively during good months, and build multiple income streams."

Your practical planning toolkit

Accommodation request template:

Dear [HR/Manager],

I am writing to request reasonable accommodations under the [relevant law]. I have a chronic medical condition that occasionally affects my work performance.

Proposed accommodations:

1. [Specific request with business justification]
2. [Second request with minimal business impact]
3. [Third request with productivity benefit]

These accommodations would enable me to maintain my strong performance while managing my health condition. I'm happy to discuss alternatives that meet both my medical needs and business requirements.

I've attached medical documentation confirming my need for accommodations. Please let me know the next steps in your process.

Sincerely, [Your name]

Relationship check-in worksheet:

Monthly with partner:

- How supported do you feel? (1-10)
- What worked well this month?
- What created stress?
- Upcoming challenges?
- Intimacy satisfaction?
- Support needed?

Financial tracking essentials:

- Medical expenses (every copay, medication, supply)
- Mileage to appointments
- Lost wages documentation
- Insurance EOBs organized
- HSA/FSA receipts
- Accommodation costs

Benefits application checklist:

- Complete work history
- Medical records (all providers)
- Treatment documentation
- Functional capacity evaluations

- Mental health records
- Daily activity logs
- Third-party statements

Building a life that works with endometriosis

Here's the truth: endometriosis will impact your work, education, relationships, and finances. That's not pessimism—it's reality. But impact doesn't mean destruction.

The women who thrive with endometriosis aren't the ones with mild symptoms. They're the ones who stopped apologizing for their needs, learned their rights, built support systems, and created lives that accommodate their reality instead of fighting it.

"I spent five years trying to pretend endometriosis didn't affect my life," reflects Nicole. "Once I accepted it did—and deserved accommodations—everything changed. My career improved because I wasn't constantly struggling. My marriage strengthened because we stopped pretending everything was fine. My friendships deepened because I let people actually help."

Chapter 10 awaits, where we'll look at research breakthroughs and future hope. But your future starts with decisions you make today about work, school, relationships, and finances. You have rights. You have options. You have value beyond your productivity.

Endometriosis might be part of your story, but it doesn't get to write the ending.

Chapter 10:Research and Hope

The notification popped up on my phone during another sleepless 3 AM endometriosis session. "New clinical trial for endometriosis—recruiting now." Six months earlier, I would have scrolled past. Been there, tried that, got the disappointment t-shirt. But something made me click.

That click led to my enrollment in a trial for a completely new class of medication—one that didn't mess with hormones, didn't cause menopause, didn't require surgery. Two years later, I'm not cured (let's stay realistic), but I'm living with 70% less pain and zero side effects.

Here's what that taught me: while we've been fighting our daily battles with endometriosis, researchers have been quietly revolutionizing the field. The next five years will bring more advancement than the previous fifty. Not empty promises—real, funded, in-progress change.

The research explosion nobody saw coming

Something shifted in endometriosis research around 2023. Suddenly, major institutions started taking it seriously. The National Institute of Child Health and Human Development launched the ACT ENDO Initiative—Advancing Clinical Trials in Endometriosis—with unprecedented funding and scope.

"We're not tweaking existing treatments anymore," explains Dr. Rebecca Martinez, who leads one of the funded studies. "We're completely rethinking endometriosis. Is it autoimmune? Metabolic? Infectious? All of the above? Once you ask different questions, you get different answers."

The numbers blow my mind: 387 active clinical trials for endometriosis as of 2024. Five years ago? Maybe 50. The pipeline includes:

- Non-hormonal pain medications targeting specific inflammatory pathways
- Medications that prevent lesion formation without affecting fertility
- Diagnostic blood tests that could replace surgery
- Treatments addressing the gut-brain-endometrium connection
- Gene therapy approaches for severe cases

But here's what really excites me—the integration of **artificial intelligence**. AI systems now detect endometriosis lesions during surgery with 97.57% accuracy, catching disease human eyes miss. Imagine: no more "we didn't find anything" when you wake up from diagnostic surgery.

Dr. Chen's team at Stanford developed an AI that predicts endometriosis from standard pelvic MRIs—previously thought impossible. "The AI sees patterns in tissue density and inflammation that radiologists can't detect. We're essentially teaching computers to diagnose what doctors have missed for decades".

The microbiome connection changes everything

Plot twist: your gut bacteria might be running the endometriosis show. Research exploded showing women with endometriosis have distinctly different microbiomes—not just in their gut, but in their reproductive tract.

This isn't "take probiotics and call me in the morning" simplicity. We're talking about specific bacterial strains that either promote or protect against endometriosis. Some produce inflammatory compounds. Others manufacture protective short-chain fatty acids.

Lisa participated in a microbiome modulation trial: "They analyzed my gut bacteria, identified problem strains, and used targeted prebiotics and specific probiotic strains to shift the balance. My bloating disappeared first. Then my pain levels dropped. It felt like science fiction, but it worked."

Companies are developing "endometriosis-specific" probiotic formulations based on this research. Unlike generic probiotics, these target the exact dysbiosis patterns found in endometriosis patients. Early results show 40-60% symptom improvement in combination with standard treatment.

Patient advocacy rewrites the rules

While scientists worked in labs, patients revolutionized advocacy. The **#1in10 movement** generated over 15,000 social media posts in 2024 alone, forcing endometriosis into mainstream conversation.

"We stopped being polite about period pain," says Samantha Chen, who started the viral TikTok series "Endometriosis Reality Check." "When millions of women share their stories simultaneously, people can't ignore us anymore."

Celebrity advocacy amplified patient voices. When soccer star Megan Rapinoe revealed her endometriosis struggle, youth sports leagues worldwide started taking menstrual health seriously. Actress Padma Lakshmi's advocacy led to endometriosis education in New York schools. Each famous voice gives permission for millions to speak up.

But the real victory? **Policy changes**. The CARE Act (Comprehensive Assistance for Relief of Endometriosis), proposed in Congress, would allocate $50 million annually for research and education. States are passing laws requiring endometriosis education in medical schools. Insurance companies face pressure to cover excision surgery.

"We're not begging anymore," states Maria Rodriguez, who testified before Congress. "We're demanding. There's a difference."

Building your modern support network

The isolation of chronic illness met its match in digital connection. Reddit's r/endometriosis and r/Endo communities generated over 30,000 posts in 2024, creating a 24/7 support network.

But here's the thing—online support varies wildly in quality. Use this framework:

Green flag communities:

- Diverse voices and experiences
- Evidence-based information sharing
- Celebration of all treatment choices
- Active moderation against misinformation
- Support without toxic positivity

Red flag spaces:

- One-size-fits-all treatment pushing
- Shaming medication or surgical choices
- Competitive suffering ("my pain is worse")
- Unverified "cures" promoted
- Negativity without hope

"I found my surgery buddy through Reddit," shares Ashley. "We had surgery the same week, texted through recovery, compared notes. Having someone who 'got it' made everything bearable."

Local support groups offer different benefits—real hugs, shared doctors, carpool to appointments. Finding them:

- Hospital gynecology departments often host groups
- Endometriosis organizations list local chapters
- Facebook search "[your city] endometriosis support"
- Meetup.com chronic illness groups
- Ask your doctor—they know who organizes locally

Starting your own group? Keep it simple:

1. Pick a consistent time/place (library meeting rooms are often free)
2. Create basic ground rules (confidentiality, respect for all treatments)
3. Rotate discussion topics so it's not just venting
4. Include social elements—coffee after meetings builds real friendships
5. Stay solution-focused while validating struggles

Your professional dream team assembly

Stop looking for one perfect doctor. Build a team. Your endometriosis management might include:

- **Endometriosis specialist** (quarterback of your team)
- **Pain management physician** (not just pills—comprehensive approaches)
- **Pelvic floor physical therapist** (absolutely essential)
- **Mental health provider** specializing in chronic illness
- **Nutritionist** understanding inflammatory conditions
- **Acupuncturist** or massage therapist for complementary care

"I spent years doctor-shopping for 'the one,'" reflects Carmen. "Now I have a team. My surgeon handles surgery. My pain doc manages medications. My therapist keeps me sane. My PT keeps me functional. Together, they're incredible."

Team coordination tips:

- Sign releases so they can communicate
- Keep central records you control
- Brief each provider on what others are doing
- Don't let ego battles affect your care
- You're the CEO of your health team

Creating your personalized action plan

After ten chapters of information, you need a framework for action. Not a rigid plan—endometriosis laughs at rigid plans—but a flexible guide.

Your 3-month sprint goals:

- Pick ONE symptom to focus on improving
- Implement TWO new management strategies
- Schedule THREE overdue appointments
- Track progress in a simple system
- Celebrate small wins

"I tried to overhaul everything at once," admits Patricia. "Total failure. Then I focused just on improving sleep for three months. That success motivated the next change."

6-month milestone mapping:

- Evaluate what's working/not working
- Adjust treatment plan based on data
- Address one lifestyle factor thoroughly
- Build support system intentionally
- Plan for seasonal symptom changes

Annual revolution review:

- Comprehensive health assessment
- Insurance and financial planning
- Career/education adjustments needed
- Relationship status and needs
- Quality of life honest evaluation

When to pivot strategies

Endometriosis changes. Your management needs to change too. Pivot when:

- Current treatment plateaus after 6 months
- Side effects outweigh benefits
- Life circumstances shift significantly
- New treatments become available
- Your priorities change (fertility, career, etc.)

"I stayed on birth control for three years past when it stopped helping," shares Rachel. "I was afraid to change. But pivoting to different management opened up my life again."

Hope anchored in reality

Let me be clear: we're not getting a cure next year. Or probably next decade. But—and this is a massive but—we're getting better treatments, faster diagnosis, more understanding, and actual respect.

Success with endometriosis needs redefinition:

- Perfect health? Probably not
- Significantly reduced symptoms? Absolutely possible
- Normal life between flares? Achievable
- Career and relationships? Adaptable but viable
- Joy and meaning? 100% available

"I mourned my pre-endometriosis life for years," reflects Diana. "Then I realized—this life, with its challenges and adaptations, taught me resilience I never knew I had. I wouldn't choose endometriosis, but I'm proud of who it's made me become."

Your manifesto for moving forward

Write this. Seriously. Put pen to paper and create your personal endometriosis manifesto:

"I have endometriosis. It's part of my story but not my identity.

I deserve comprehensive medical care and will advocate until I get it.

I release guilt about what I cannot do and celebrate what I can.

I surround myself with people who support my reality.

I make decisions based on my values, not others' expectations.

I stay informed about research but don't chase every new treatment.

I define success by my own standards.

I choose hope without denying difficulty."

Add your own truths. Read it on hard days. Update it as you grow.

The research participation opportunity

Want to be part of the solution? Clinical trials need participants. Here's how:

1. Search ClinicalTrials.gov for endometriosis studies

2. Filter by location and eligibility
3. Understand different trial phases:
    o Phase 1: Safety testing (higher risk, closer monitoring)
    o Phase 2: Effectiveness testing (moderate risk)
    o Phase 3: Comparison to standard treatment (lower risk)
4. Ask about compensation, travel reimbursement, and care coverage
5. Never feel obligated—you can leave any trial anytime

"Participating in research gave me purpose," shares Monica. "My pain contributed to potentially helping millions. That meaning made the hard days easier."

Your tomorrow starts today

As we close not just this chapter but this entire exploration of endometriosis, I want to leave you with this: you're living through the most hopeful time in endometriosis history.

Yes, you're still in pain. Yes, the system still fails us. Yes, some days feel impossible. All true.

Also true: researchers finally listen. Treatments finally advance. Doctors finally learn. Patients finally unite. Change finally comes.

Your part? Keep going. Keep advocating. Keep connecting. Keep hoping. Not because everything's fine—it's not. But because you deserve every advancement coming, and they ARE coming.

The woman who clicked on that clinical trial notification at 3 AM? She's writing this conclusion pain-free for the first time in fifteen years. Not cured. Not perfect. But proof that persistence pays off.

Your story isn't over. It's just getting interesting.

Turn the page. The appendices await with every practical resource you need. Then close this book and open your next chapter—armed with knowledge, supported by community, and ready for whatever comes next.

Because endometriosis might be chronic, but so is your strength.

And that, my friend, makes all the difference.

References

1. **NICE** 2024. *Endometriosis: diagnosis and management (NG73).* Available at: https://www.nice.org.uk/guidance/ng73 (Accessed 2 June 2025). (NICE)

2. **Becker, C.M.** *et al.* 2022. 'ESHRE guideline: endometriosis'. *Human Reproduction Open*, 2022(2), hoac009. Available at: https://academic.oup.com/hropen/article/2022/2/hoac009/6537540 (Accessed 18 July 2025). (Oxford Academic)

3. **Zondervan, K.T., Becker, C.M. & Missmer, S.A.** 2020. 'Endometriosis'. *New England Journal of Medicine*, 382(13), 1244–1256. Available at: https://www.nejm.org/doi/full/10.1056/NEJMra1810764 (Accessed 23 Aug 2025). (New England Journal of Medicine)

4. **Zondervan, K.T.** *et al.* 2018. 'Endometriosis'. *Nature Reviews Disease Primers*, 4, 9. Available at: https://www.nature.com/articles/s41572-018-0008-5 (Accessed 11 July 2025). (Nature)

5. **Bafort, C.** *et al.* 2020. 'Laparoscopic surgery for endometriosis'. *Cochrane Database of Systematic Reviews*, CD011031. Available at: https://www.cochranelibrary.com/cdsr/doi/10.1002/14651858.CD011031.pub3/full (Accessed 18 June 2025). (Cochrane Library)

6. **Nisenblat, V.** *et al.* 2016. 'Blood biomarkers for the non-invasive diagnosis of endometriosis'. *Cochrane Database of Systematic Reviews*, 2016(5), CD012179. Available at: https://pubmed.ncbi.nlm.nih.gov/27132058/ (Accessed 17 July 2025). (PubMed)

7. **Guerriero, S.** *et al.* 2016. 'Systematic approach to sonographic evaluation of the pelvis in women with suspected endometriosis (IDEA consensus)'. *Ultrasound in Obstetrics & Gynecology*, 48(3), 318–332. Available at: https://obgyn.onlinelibrary.wiley.com/doi/full/10.1002/uog.15955 (Accessed 15 Aug 2025). (Obstetrics & Gynecology)

8. **Harmsen, M.J.** *et al.* 2022. 'Consensus on revised definitions of MUSA features of adenomyosis'. *Ultrasound in Obstetrics & Gynecology*, 59(4), 496–507. Available at: https://obgyn.onlinelibrary.wiley.com/doi/10.1002/uog.24786 (Accessed 20 June 2025). (Obstetrics & Gynecology)

9. **Thomassin-Naggara, I.** *et al.* 2025. 'ESUR consensus MRI for endometriosis—indications, reporting and classifications'. *European Radiology*. Available at: https://pubmed.ncbi.nlm.nih.gov/40425757/ (Accessed 14 July 2025). (PubMed)

10. **Quesada, J.** *et al.* 2023. 'Endometriosis: a multimodal imaging review'. *European Journal of Radiology*, 162, 110734. Available at: https://www.ejradiology.com/article/S0720-048X%2822%2900460-0/fulltext (Accessed 14 June 2025).

11. **Keckstein, J.** *et al.* 2021. 'The #Enzian classification of endometriosis (2021 revision)'. *Acta Obstetricia et Gynecologica Scandinavica*, 100(7), 1165–1175. Available at: https://obgyn.onlinelibrary.wiley.com/doi/abs/10.1111/aogs.14099 (Accessed 13 Aug 2025).

12. **Johnson, N.P.** *et al.* 2017. 'World Endometriosis Society consensus on the classification of endometriosis'. *Human Reproduction*, 32(2), 315–324. Available at: https://academic.oup.com/humrep/article/32/2/315/26313 90 (Accessed 1 July 2025).

13. **Vermeulen, N.** *et al.* 2021. 'Endometriosis classification, staging and reporting systems: a review...'. *Human Reproduction Open*, 2021(4), hoab025. Available at: https://pubmed.ncbi.nlm.nih.gov/34693032/ (Accessed 20 Aug 2025).

14. **Adamson, G.D. & Pasta, D.J.** 2010. 'Endometriosis Fertility Index: the new, validated staging system'. *Fertility and Sterility*, 94(5), 1609–1615. Available at: https://pubmed.ncbi.nlm.nih.gov/19931076/ (Accessed 2 June 2025).

15. **Tomassetti, C.** *et al.* 2013. 'External validation of the Endometriosis Fertility Index (EFI)'. *Human Reproduction*, 28(5), 1280–1288. Available at: https://academic.oup.com/humrep/article/28/5/1280/9405 39 (Accessed 20 Aug 2025).

16. **Nnoaham, K.E.** *et al.* 2011. 'Impact of endometriosis on quality of life and work productivity'. *Fertility and Sterility*, 96(2), 366–373.e8. Available at: https://pubmed.ncbi.nlm.nih.gov/21718982/ (Accessed 20 Aug 2025).

17. **Ballard, K.** *et al.* 2006. 'What's the delay? A qualitative study of women's experience of reaching a diagnosis of endometriosis'. *Fertility and Sterility*, 86(5), 1296–1301. Available at: https://pubmed.ncbi.nlm.nih.gov/17070183/ (Accessed 2 July 2025).

18. **Pearce, C.L.** *et al.* 2012. 'Association between endometriosis and risk of histological subtypes of

ovarian cancer'. *The Lancet Oncology*, 13(4), 385–394. Available at: https://pubmed.ncbi.nlm.nih.gov/22361336/ (Accessed 17 Aug 2025).

19. **Brilhante, A.V.M.** *et al.* 2017. 'Endometriosis and ovarian cancer: an integrative review'. *Clinical Ovarian and Other Gynecologic Cancer*, 10(1), 21–26. Available at: https://pmc.ncbi.nlm.nih.gov/articles/PMC5563086/ (Accessed 16 June 2025).

20. **Taylor, H.S.** *et al.* 2017. 'Treatment of endometriosis-associated pain with elagolix, an oral GnRH antagonist'. *New England Journal of Medicine*, 377(1), 28–40. Available at: https://www.nejm.org/doi/full/10.1056/NEJMoa1700089 (Accessed 18 Aug 2025)

21. **Giudice, L.C.** *et al.* 2022. 'Once-daily oral relugolix combination therapy versus placebo in endometriosis-associated pain (SPIRIT 1 & 2)'. *The Lancet*, 399(10343), 2267–2279. Available at: https://www.thelancet.com/journals/lancet/article/PIIS0140-6736%2822%2900622-5/fulltext (Accessed 16 Aug 2025).

22. **NICE** 2021. *Chronic pain in over 16s: assessment and management (NG193)*. Available at: https://www.nice.org.uk/guidance/ng193 (Accessed 12 July 2025).

23. **Guerriero, S.** *et al.* 2024. 'Addendum to the IDEA consensus: sonographic assessment of the parametrium'. *Ultrasound in Obstetrics & Gynecology*, 64(2), 275–280. Available at: https://obgyn.onlinelibrary.wiley.com/doi/10.1002/uog.27558 (Accessed 16 July 2025).

24. **Condous, G.** *et al.* 2024. 'Non-invasive imaging techniques for diagnosis of pelvic deep endometriosis and endometriosis classification systems: International Consensus Statement'. *Journal of Minimally Invasive Gynecology*, 31(7), 557–573. Available at: https://pubmed.ncbi.nlm.nih.gov/38808587/ (Accessed 2 Aug 2025).

25. **Hirsch, M.** *et al.* 2018. 'Diagnosis and management of endometriosis: a systematic review of international and national guidelines'. *BJOG*, 125(5), 556–564. Available at: https://pubmed.ncbi.nlm.nih.gov/28755422/ (Accessed 10 Aug 2025).

www.ingramcontent.com/pod-product-compliance
Lightning Source LLC
Chambersburg PA
CBHW071230290326
41931CB00037B/2616